A Pocket Reference for Psychiatrists

A Pocket Reference for Psychiatrists

Susan C. Jenkins, M.D.
Research Fellow in Psychiatry, Mayo Graduate School of Medicine, Rochester, Minnesota

Timothy P. Gibbs, M.D.
Resident in Child and Adolescent Psychiatry, Mayo Graduate School of Medicine, Rochester, Minnesota

Sally R. Szymanski, D.O.
Senior Resident in Psychiatry, Mayo Graduate School of Medicine, Rochester, Minnesota

With Contributors

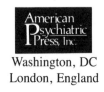
American Psychiatric Press, Inc.

Washington, DC
London, England

Copyright 1990 Mayo Foundation
ALL RIGHTS RESERVED
Manufactured in the United States of America
94 93   5 4
First Edition

American Psychiatric Press, Inc.
1400 K Street, N.W.
Washington, DC 20005

The paper used in this publication meets the minimum requirements
of the American National Standard for Information Sciences—Per-
manence of Paper for Printed Library Materials, ANSI Z39.48-
1984.

Library of Congress Cataloging-in-Publication Data

A pocket reference for psychiatrists / by Susan C. Jenkins,
    Timothy P. Gibbs, Sally R. Szymanski.—1st ed.
        p.   cm.
    ISBN 0-88048-109-9 (alk. paper)
    1. Mental illness—Diagnosis—Handbooks, manuals,
  etc.   2. Mental illness—Chemotherapy—Handbooks, manuals,
  etc.   3. Psychotropic drugs—Handbooks, manuals,
  etc.   I. Jenkins, Susan C., 1955-   .
II. Gibbs, Timothy P., 1955-   . III. Szymanski, Sally R.
    [DNLM: 1. Mental Disorders—diagnosis—handbooks.
    2. Mental Disorders—therapy—handbooks.   3. Psychotropic
Drugs—handbooks.
WM 34 P7391
RC469.P57   1990
616.89—dc20
DNLM/DLC
for Library of Congress   90-276
                                                              CIP

British Library Cataloguing in Publication Data

A CIP record is available from the British Library.

Dr. Jenkins is currently Consulting Psychiatrist, Associates in Psychiatry and Psychology, Rochester, Minnesota.

Dr. Gibbs is currently Staff Child and Adolescent Psychiatrist, Minneapolis Psychiatric Institute; Chairperson, Sub-Section of Child and Adolescent Psychiatry, Abbott-Northwestern Hospital; Minneapolis, Minnesota.

Dr. Szymanski is currently Research Psychiatrist, Department of Psychiatric Research, Hillside Hospital, Long Island Jewish Medical Center, Glen Oaks, New York.

CONTENTS

GENERAL DIAGNOSTIC INFORMATION

ADDITIONAL CONTRIBUTORS

ELLIOTT RICHELSON, M.D.

Director for Research, Mayo Clinic Jacksonville, Jacksonville, Florida; Professor of Psychiatry and Professor of Pharmacology, Mayo Medical School, Rochester, Minnesota

MARK R. HANSEN, M.D.

Consultant, Department of Psychiatry and Psychology, Mayo Clinic and Mayo Foundation; Assistant Professor of Psychiatry, Mayo Medical School; Rochester, Minnesota

ROBERT C. COLLIGAN, Ph.D.

Head, Section of Psychology, Mayo Clinic and Mayo Foundation; Professor of Psychology, Mayo Medical School; Rochester, Minnesota

NOTICE TO READERS

This material is intended as a memory aid only. In no case should physicians rely upon this handbook as the sole source of information for prescribing drugs or for making decisions about patient care. Physicians are referred to standard psychiatry textbooks, *Physicians' Desk Reference, Drug Information* by the American Hospital Formulary Service, and drug package inserts for more complete diagnostic and treatment information.

Statutes regarding restraints, electroconvulsive therapy, drug testing, and other issues vary among states and treatment settings and are subject to revision. Physicians are responsible for becoming familiar with current law in their area of practice.

PREFACE

A Pocket Reference for Psychiatrists is a compendium of tables and lists to be used by persons already familiar with psychiatry. We have included information that is too detailed to be recalled with certainty but which is necessary in the daily practice of psychiatry. Also included are lists that the clinician will find to be useful reminders in evaluation and treatment. Although the book was designed specifically for use by psychiatrists, our experience has shown that medical students, residents, family practitioners, nurses, psychologists, social workers, and other mental health professionals will also find it useful.

The book was conceived as the editors progressed through their residency training. We found available house officer guides too wordy for rapid reference and sometimes lacking key data needed in a clinical setting. Textbooks were more detailed but too cumbersome for ward use. We began designing the type of handbook we wished we had. We collected tables and lists from journals, textbooks, and handouts. In many cases, available sources did not present the material in a succinct format and we devised our own tables. A manuscript was prepared, edited, and distributed to the psychiatry staff and residents at the Mayo Clinic where it was "field-tested" for 2 years. The suggestions of many professionals who read and used the book were incorporated in the present edition.

The book is organized into sections pertaining to the General Interview and Diagnosis, Specialized Interviews, Psychological Assessment, Medical Psychiatry, Psychopharmacology, and Electroconvulsive Therapy. Psychotherapies and theories of personality development and psychopathology are not included here. Although this information is of major importance in psychiatric practice, it does not lend itself well to this type of format, and once mastered, psychoanalytic and psychotherapeutic principles are not quickly forgotten.

Information was included because of its clinical utility and the need for easy access in the clinical setting. To retain the convenience of a pocket reference, each subject is presented only briefly and often in a tabular or list-type format. The reader is assumed to be familiar with the rudiments of psychiatric interview and diagnosis. For example, although side effects of psychopharmacologic agents are presented, their therapeutic indications are not. The reader may wish to consult a comprehensive text or one of the listed references for more information.

No book of this type is ever complete. We all have different memory lacunae and psychiatry is rapidly changing. Readers are encouraged to use blank pages and margin spaces to refine tables to their liking.

Our thanks to the staff and residents of the Mayo Clinic Department of Psychiatry and Psychology who offered advice and encouragement in the preparation of this handbook. Special acknowledgments are due the following people: John L. Black, M.D., John E. Huxsahl, M.D., and Teresa A. Rummans, M.D., for suggestions on the initial project; Steven I. Altchuler, M.D., Ph.D., Paul A. Fredrickson, M.D., Sheila G. Jowsey, M.D., Eric K. Milliner, M.D., Robert M. Morse, M.D., Thomas P. Moyer, Ph.D., Ronald Neeper, Ph.D., Douglas A. Nichols, M.D., Jarrett W. Richardson, M.D., and Mark S. Schwartz, Ph.D., for knowledgeable assistance in preparing some sections of the material; Carol L. Kornblith, Ph.D., for editing the manuscript; Theresa A. Funk and Dianne F. Kemp for preparation of the manuscript; and Patricia J. Calvert for proofreading the manuscript. We thank Gordon L. Moore, M.D., and Maurice J. Martin, M.D., for their support and sponsorship of this project. The editors and reviewers at the American Psychiatric Press, Inc., provided valuable professional criticism. Particular appreciation is due our contributors: Elliott Richelson, M.D., for permission to use his data on neurotransmitter affinities and consultation regarding the many psychopharmacology tables; Robert C. Colligan, Ph.D., for his enthusiastic moral support and assistance with preparation of the psychology section; and Mark R. Hansen, M.D., who worked with us through several revisions of this manuscript.

Susan C. Jenkins, M.D.

GENERAL DIAGNOSTIC INFORMATION

PSYCHIATRIC HISTORY

CLINICAL EVALUATION

Identification
Chief complaint
Source of information
History of present illness (include current level of functioning)
Past psychiatric history (include previous somatic treatments and psychotherapy)
Past medical history (include current treatment)
Family medical history (include psychiatric disorders and substance abuse)
Social and developmental history*
Review of systems*
Mental status examination*
Physical examination
Laboratory examination*
Impression (include DSM-III-R differential diagnosis if known)
    Document potential for self-injury or violence
Plan
    Document severity of illness and intensity of care required

SOCIAL AND DEVELOPMENTAL HISTORY

Childhood
    Developmental milestones   Early trauma
    Earliest memories   Sexual development
    Childhood temperament   Transition out of home

*Further information presented later in this book.

SOCIAL AND DEVELOPMENTAL HISTORY—continued

Family of Origin
    Relation to parents   Home stability
    Relation to siblings   Method of discipline
Institutional History
    Education   Legal problems
    Military experience   Marriage
    Employment
Current Social Setting
    Living quarters   Drug or alcohol use
    Family   Financial status
    Occupation   Hobbies
    Peer relations   Habits
    Religion
Other
    Most pleasant/   Fears
       unpleasant experience   Goals
    Most influential person in life

PSYCHIATRIC REVIEW OF SYSTEMS

These major areas of information should be covered during an initial diagnostic encounter. They are best approached as they naturally arise during the interview. This is included as a checklist for interviewers.

Behavior Pattern: activity level, organization of activity, self-destructive patterns, daily routine
Somatic Disturbance: vegetative symptoms, medical complaints or problems, psychosomatic complaints
Thought Disturbance: concentration or memory disturbance, thought content, neurotic patterns, formal thought disorder
Adjustment Problems: family, friends, marriage, work, school; sexual, legal, financial, spiritual
Affective Disturbance: anger, depression, anxiety, euphoria, lability, restricted affect
Use of Drugs or Medicines: prescription, over-the-counter, or "health food" preparations; illicit drugs; caffeine, nicotine, alcohol
Potential for Violence or Suicide; Victimization or Traumatic Experiences: inquire specifically

For each of the above categories the interviewer may wish to inquire as to the onset, duration, periodicity, and intensity of the symptom. Specific symptoms are listed in the Mental Status Examination (see below).

MENTAL STATUS EXAMINATION

Information pertinent to the mental status examination is gathered throughout the patient encounter. These observations can be organized into the following format for the clinical record.

I. *Attitude, appearance, and motor activity*
   Ability to conduct interview   Eye contact
       Cooperativeness   Facies
       Reliability/completeness   Psychomotor activity
   Dress or grooming   Tremors/tics/fidgeting

II. *Mood and affect*
    Depression   Flat affect
    Anxiety   Labile affect
    Euphoria   Inappropriate affect
    Anger/hostility

III. *Structure of thought and speech*
     Structural abnormalities   Speech rate
         Incoherence   Speech production
         Blocking
         Perseveration
         Loosening of associations
         Flight of ideas
         Tangentiality
         Circumstantiality
         Distractibility
         Clang associations/rhyming/
             punning
         Neologisms

IV. *Content of thought and speech*
    Preoccupation/rumination   Grandiosity
    Somatic concern/hypochondriasis   Ideas of reference/influence
    Derealization/depersonalization   Excessive religiosity
    Compulsions/obsessions   Delusions
    Dreams and fantasies   Type(s) and content

  V. *Perception*
      Hallucinations
          Type(s) and content
      Illusions

 VI. *Sensorium and cognition*
      Orientation   Retention and recall
      Attention   Performance of commands
      Memory   Calculations
         Immediate recall   Abstractions
         Recent   General information
         Remote   Judgment
         Confabulation   Estimated intelligence

VII. *Potential for destructiveness*
      Suicide
      Violence

VIII. *Insight and motivation*
      Recognition of emotional problems
      Motivation for treatment

"Mini-Mental State"

Maximum possible score is 30.
A score of 20 or less indicates significant impairment of cognitive abilities such as is found in dementia, delirium, or major mental disorder.

Maximum Score	Score	**ORIENTATION**
5	( )	What is the: (day of the week) (year) (season) (date) (month)?
5	( )	Where are we: (state) (county) (town) (hospital) (floor).

		REGISTRATION
3	( )	Name 3 objects: 1 second to say each. Then ask the patient all 3 after you have said them. Give 1 point for each correct answer. Then repeat them until he learns all 3. Count trials and record.

Maximum
Score   Score

ATTENTION AND CALCULATION

5   ( ) Serial 7s. 1 point for each correct. Stop after 5 answers. Alternatively spell "world" backwards.

RECALL

3   ( ) Ask for the 3 objects repeated above. Give 1 point for each correct.

LANGUAGE

9   ( ) Name a pencil and a watch (2 points)
Repeat the following: "No ifs, ands or buts." (1 point)
Follow a 3-stage command:
   "Take a paper in your right hand, fold it in half, and put it on the floor" (3 points)
Read and obey the following:
   CLOSE YOUR EYES (1 point)
Write a sentence (1 point)
Copy design (intersecting pentagons) (1 point)

_____ **Total score**
ASSESS level of consciousness along a continuum: Alert, Drowsy, Stupor, Coma.

From Folstein MF, Folstein SE, McHugh PR: "Mini-mental state": a practical method for grading the cognitive state of patients for the clinician. J Psychiatr Res 12:189–198, 1975. By permission of Pergamon Press.
See also: Kokmen E, Naessens JM, Offord KP: A short test of mental status: description and preliminary results. Mayo Clin Proc 62:281–288, 1987.

Cognitive Mental Status Examination Items

The following items may be used in mental status examinations. Clinicians may write their own items in the margins.

1. Orientation—Name, date, location of interview, and purpose of interview

2. Attention/retention/recall—Four unrelated words:
   1. Apple   2. Dishwasher   3. Pride   4. Tractor

   Three items:
   1. Red book   2. Silver pencil   3. Spotted pony

3. Immediate recall/concentration—Digit span (random digits):

4-3	4-1
2-5-4	3-2-6
7-8-3-2	8-1-7-5
4-1-7-3-5	4-0-3-6-8
6-2-7-5-8-3	0-8-6-2-4-5
1-6-7-9-4-5-0	9-6-7-8-2-1-3
5-0-8-7-9-6-3-4	7-1-6-8-3-0-9-2
1-3-2-6-8-7-5-4-0	7-3-1-0-4-2-5-8-6

4. Performance of commands
   Point to my shoe
   Show me your teeth
   Put your left hand on your right ear

5. Concentration/calculation: Serial 7s
                                Simple arithmetic

6. Ability to abstract

   Proverbs:
   Don't cry over spilled milk.
   A stitch in time saves nine.
   You can't judge a book by its cover.
   Rome wasn't built in a day.
   People who live in glass houses shouldn't throw stones.
   A golden hammer breaks an iron door.
   Similarities: Orange-Apple
                   Dog-Cat
                   Fly-Tree

7. General knowledge/recall: Presidents
                                   Capitals of Europe
                                   Capitals of states

8. Judgment:
    What would you do if you found a wallet with some important-looking papers in it, but no money?
    What would you do if you were in a room and the curtains caught on fire?
    What would you do if you were lost in the city?

DSM-III-R CLASSIFICATION

AXES I AND II CATEGORIES AND CODES

All official DSM-III-R codes are included in ICD-9-CM. Codes followed by an * are used for more than one DSM-III-R diagnosis or subtype in order to maintain compatibility with ICD-9-CM.

A long dash following a diagnostic term indicates the need for a fifth digit subtype or other qualifying term.

The term *specify* following the name of some diagnostic categories indicates qualifying terms that clinicians may wish to add in parentheses after the name of the disorder.

NOS = Not Otherwise
           Specified

The current severity of a disorder may be specified after the diagnosis as:

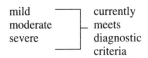

mild   currently
moderate   meets
severe   diagnostic
                  criteria

in partial remission
   (or residual state)
in complete remission

DISORDERS USUALLY FIRST EVIDENT IN INFANCY, CHILDHOOD, OR ADOLESCENCE

DEVELOPMENTAL DISORDERS
Note: These are coded on Axis II.

Mental Retardation
317.00　Mild mental retardation
318.00　Moderate mental retardation
318.10　Severe mental retardation
318.20　Profound mental retardation
319.00　Unspecified mental retardation

Pervasive Developmental Disorders
299.00　Autistic disorder
　　　　　Specify if childhood onset
299.80　Pervasive developmental disorder NOS

Specific Developmental Disorders

Academic skills disorders
315.10　Developmental arithmetic disorder
315.80　Developmental expressive writing disorder
315.00　Developmental reading disorder

Language and speech disorders
315.39　Developmental articulation disorder
315.31*Developmental expressive language disorder
315.31*Developmental receptive language disorder

Motor skills disorders
315.40　Developmental coordination disorder
315.90*Specific developmental disorder NOS

Other Developmental Disorders
315.90*Developmental disorder NOS

Disruptive Behavior Disorders
314.01　Attention-deficit hyperactivity disorder

　　　　　Conduct disorder,
312.20　group type
312.00　solitary aggressive type
312.90　undifferentiated type
313.81　Oppositional defiant disorder

Anxiety Disorders of Childhood or Adolescence
309.21　Separation anxiety disorder
313.21　Avoidant disorder of childhood or adolescence
313.00　Overanxious disorder

Eating Disorders
307.10　Anorexia nervosa
307.51　Bulimia nervosa
307.52　Pica
307.53　Rumination disorder of infancy
307.50　Eating disorder NOS

Gender Identity Disorders
302.60　Gender identity disorder of childhood
302.50　Transsexualism
　　　　　Specify sexual history: asexual, homosexual, heterosexual, unspecified

302.85*Gender identity disorder of adolescence or adulthood, nontrans-sexual type
Specify sexual history: asexual, homosexual, heterosexual, unspecified

302.85*Gender identity disorder NOS

Tic Disorders
307.23 Tourette's disorder
307.22 Chronic motor or vocal tic disorder
307.21 Transient tic disorder
Specify: single episode or recurrent
307.20 Tic disorder NOS

Elimination Disorders
307.70 Functional encopresis
Specify: primary or secondary type
307.60 Functional enuresis
Specify: primary or secondary type
Specify: nocturnal only, diurnal only, nocturnal and diurnal

Speech Disorders Not Elsewhere Classified
307.00* Cluttering
307.00* Stuttering

Other Disorders of Infancy, Childhood, or Adolescence
313.23 Elective mutism
313.82 Identity disorder

313.89 Reactive attachment disorder of infancy or early childhood
307.30 Stereotypy/habit disorder
314.00 Undifferentiated attention-deficit disorder

ORGANIC MENTAL DISORDERS

Dementias Arising in the Senium and Presenium
Primary degenerative dementia of the Alzheimer type, senile onset,
290.30 with delirium
290.20 with delusions
290.21 with depression
290.00* uncomplicated
(Note: code 331.00 Alzheimer's disease on Axis III)

Code in fifth digit:
1 = with delirium, 2 = with delusions, 3 = with depression, 0* = uncomplicated
290.1x Primary degenerative dementia of the Alzheimer type, presenile onset, _____
(Note: code 331.00 Alzheimer's disease on Axis III)
290.4x Multi-infarct dementia, _____
290.00* Senile dementia NOS
Specify etiology on Axis III if known

290.10*Presenile dementia
NOS

> *Specify* etiology on
> Axis III if known
> (e.g., Pick's disease,
> Jakob-Creutzfeldt
> disease)

**Psychoactive
Substance–Induced
Organic Mental Disorders**

Alcohol
303.00 intoxication
291.40 idiosyncratic intoxication
291.80 Uncomplicated alcohol
withdrawal
291.00 withdrawal delirium
291.30 hallucinosis
291.10 amnestic disorder
291.20 Dementia associated
with alcoholism

Amphetamine or simi-
larly acting sympatho-
mimetic
305.70* intoxication
292.00* withdrawal
292.81* delirium
292.11* delusional disorder

Caffeine
305.90* intoxication

Cannabis
305.20* intoxication
292.11* delusional disorder

Cocaine
305.60* intoxication
292.00* withdrawal
292.81* delirium
292.11* delusional disorder

Hallucinogen
305.30* hallucinosis
292.11* delusional disorder

292.84* mood disorder
292.89*Posthallucinogen
perception disorder

Inhalant
305.90*intoxication

Nicotine
292.00*withdrawal

Opioid
305.50*intoxication
292.00*withdrawal

Phencyclidine (PCP) or
similarly acting
arylcyclohexylamine
305.90*intoxication
292.81*delirium
292.11*delusional disorder
292.84*mood disorder
292.90*organic mental disorder
NOS

Sedative, hypnotic, or
anxiolytic
305.40*intoxication
292.00*Uncomplicated sedative, hypnotic, or anx-
iolytic withdrawal
292.00* withdrawal delirium
292.83*amnestic disorder

Other or unspecified
psychoactive substance
305.90*intoxication
292.00* withdrawal
292.81* delirium
292.82* dementia
292.83* amnestic disorder
292.11* delusional disorder
292.12 hallucinosis
292.84* mood disorder
292.89* anxiety disorder
292.89* personality disorder
292.90* organic mental disorder
NOS

Organic Mental Disorders Associated With Axis III Physical Disorders or Conditions, or Whose Etiology Is Unknown

293.00 Delirium
294.10 Dementia
294.00 Amnestic disorder
293.81 Organic delusional disorder
293.82 Organic hallucinosis
293.83 Organic mood disorder
        Specify: manic, depressed, mixed
294.80* Organic anxiety disorder
310.10 Organic personality disorder
        Specify if explosive type
294.80* Organic mental disorder NOS

PSYCHOACTIVE SUBSTANCE USE DISORDERS

        Alcohol
303.90 dependence
305.00 abuse
        Amphetamine or similarly acting sympathomimetic
304.40 dependence
305.70* abuse
        Cannabis
304.30 dependence
305.20* abuse
        Cocaine
304.20 dependence
305.60* abuse
        Hallucinogen
304.50* dependence
305.30* abuse
        Inhalant
304.60 dependence
305.90* abuse
        Nicotine
305.10 dependence
        Opioid
304.00 dependence
305.50* abuse
        Phencyclidine (PCP) or similarly acting arylcyclohexylamine
304.50* dependence
305.90* abuse
        Sedative, hypnotic, or anxiolytic
304.10 dependence
305.40* abuse
304.90* Polysubstance dependence
304.90* Psychoactive substance dependence NOS
305.90* Psychoactive substance abuse NOS

SCHIZOPHRENIA

Code in fifth digit:
1 = subchronic, 2 = chronic, 3 = subchronic with acute exacerbation, 4 = chronic with acute exacerbation, 5 = in remission, 0 = unspecified

        Schizophrenia,
295.2x catatonic, _____
295.1x disorganized, _____
295.3x paranoid, _____
        Specify if stable type
295.9x undifferentiated,_____

295.6x residual, _____
          Specify if late onset

DELUSIONAL (PARANOID) DISORDER

297.10 Delusional (Paranoid)
        disorder
        Specify type:
             erotomanic
             grandiose
             jealous
             persecutory
             somatic
             unspecified

PSYCHOTIC DISORDERS NOT ELSEWHERE CLASSIFIED

298.80 Brief reactive
        psychosis
295.40 Schizophreniform
        disorder
             Specify: without
             good prognostic fea-
             tures or with good
             prognostic features
295.70 Schizoaffective
        disorder
             Specify: bipolar type
             or depressive type
297.30 Induced psychotic
        disorder
298.90 Psychotic disorder
        NOS (Atypical
        psychosis)

MOOD DISORDERS

Code current state of Major Depression and Bipolar Disorder
in fifth digit:

1 = mild
2 = moderate
3 = severe, without psy-
    chotic features
4 = with psychotic features
    (*specify* mood-congruent
    or mood-incongruent)
5 = in partial remission
6 = in full remission
0 = unspecified

For major depressive episodes,
specify if chronic and *specify* if
melancholic type.

For Bipolar Disorder, Bipolar
Disorder NOS, Recurrent Major
Depression, and Depressive
Disorder NOS, *specify* if sea-
sonal pattern.

Bipolar Disorders

        Bipolar disorder,
296.6x mixed, _____
296.4x manic, _____
296.5x depressed, _____
301.13 Cyclothymia
296.70 Bipolar disorder NOS

Depressive Disorders

        Major depression,
296.2x single episode, _____
296.3x recurrent, _____
300.40 Dysthymia (or
        Depressive neurosis)
             Specify: primary or
             secondary type
             Specify: early or late
             onset
311.00 Depressive disorder
        NOS

ANXIETY DISORDERS (or Anxiety and Phobic Neuroses)

Panic disorder
- 300.21 with agoraphobia
  - *Specify* current severity of agoraphobic avoidance
  - *Specify* current severity of panic attacks
- 300.01 without agoraphobia
  - *Specify* current severity of panic attacks
- 300.22 Agoraphobia without history of panic disorder
  - *Specify* with or without limited symptom attacks
- 300.23 Social phobia
  - *Specify* if generalized type
- 300.29 Simple phobia
- 300.30 Obsessive compulsive disorder (or Obsessive compulsive neurosis)
- 309.89 Post-traumatic stress disorder
  - *Specify* if delayed onset
- 300.02 Generalized anxiety disorder
- 300.00 Anxiety disorder NOS

SOMATOFORM DISORDERS

- 300.70* Body dysmorphic disorder
- 300.11 Conversion disorder (or Hysterical neurosis, conversion type)
  - *Specify*: single episode or recurrent
- 300.70* Hypochondriasis (or Hypochondriacal neurosis)
- 300.81 Somatization disorder
- 307.80 Somatoform pain disorder
- 300.70* Undifferentiated somatoform disorder
- 300.70* Somatoform disorder NOS

DISSOCIATIVE DISORDERS (or Hysterical Neuroses, Dissociative Type)

- 300.14 Multiple personality disorder
- 300.13 Psychogenic fugue
- 300.12 Psychogenic amnesia
- 300.60 Depersonalization disorder (or Depersonalization neurosis)
- 300.15 Dissociative disorder NOS

SEXUAL DISORDERS
Paraphilias

- 302.40 Exhibitionism
- 302.81 Fetishism
- 302.89 Frotteurism
- 302.20 Pedophilia
  - *Specify*: same sex, opposite sex, same and opposite sex
  - *Specify* if limited to incest

Specify: exclusive type or nonexclusive type

302.83 Sexual masochism
302.84 Sexual sadism
302.30 Transvestic fetishism
302.82 Voyeurism
302.90* Paraphilia NOS

Sexual Dysfunctions

Specify: psychogenic only, or psychogenic and biogenic (Note: If biogenic only, code on Axis III)
Specify: lifelong or acquired
Specify: generalized or situational

Sexual desire disorders
302.71 Hypoactive sexual desire disorder
302.79 Sexual aversion disorder

Sexual arousal disorders
302.72* Female sexual arousal disorder
302.72* Male erectile disorder

Orgasm disorders
302.73 Inhibited female orgasm
302.74 Inhibited male orgasm
302.75 Premature ejaculation

Sexual pain disorders
302.76 Dyspareunia
306.51 Vaginismus
302.70 Sexual dysfunction NOS

Other Sexual Disorders
302.90* Sexual disorder NOS

SLEEP DISORDERS
Dyssomnias
Insomnia disorder
307.42* related to another mental disorder (nonorganic)
780.50* related to known organic factor
307.42* Primary insomnia
Hypersomnia disorder
307.44 related to another mental disorder (nonorganic)
780.50* related to a known organic factor
780.54 Primary hypersomnia
307.45 Sleep-wake schedule disorder
Specify: advanced or delayed phase type, disorganized type, frequently changing type
Other dyssomnias
307.40* Dyssomnia NOS

Parasomnias
307.47 Dream anxiety disorder (Nightmare disorder)
307.46* Sleep terror disorder
307.46* Sleepwalking disorder
307.40* Parasomnia NOS

FACTITIOUS DISORDERS
Factitious disorder
301.51 with physical symptoms
300.16 with psychological symptoms
300.19 Factitious disorder NOS

IMPULSE CONTROL DISORDERS NOT ELSEWHERE CLASSIFIED

312.34 Intermittent explosive disorder
312.32 Kleptomania
312.31 Pathological gambling
312.33 Pyromania
312.39* Trichotillomania
312.39* Impulse control disorder NOS

ADJUSTMENT DISORDER

Adjustment disorder
309.24 with anxious mood
309.00 with depressed mood
309.30 with disturbance of conduct
309.40 with mixed disturbance of emotions and conduct
309.28 with mixed emotional features
309.82 with physical complaints
309.83 with withdrawal
309.23 with work (or academic) inhibition
309.90 Adjustment disorder NOS

PSYCHOLOGICAL FACTORS AFFECTING PHYSICAL CONDITION

316.00 Psychological factors affecting physical condition
        Specify physical condition on Axis III

PERSONALITY DISORDERS

Note: These are coded on Axis II.

Cluster A
301.00 Paranoid
301.20 Schizoid
301.22 Schizotypal

Cluster B
301.70 Antisocial
301.83 Borderline
301.50 Histrionic
301.81 Narcissistic

Cluster C
301.82 Avoidant
301.60 Dependent
301.40 Obsessive compulsive
301.84 Passive aggressive
301.90 Personality disorder NOS

V CODES FOR CONDITIONS NOT ATTRIBUTABLE TO A MENTAL DISORDER THAT ARE A FOCUS OF ATTENTION OR TREATMENT

V62.30 Academic problem
V71.01 Adult antisocial behavior
V40.00 Borderline intellectual functioning (Note: This is coded on Axis II.)
V71.02 Childhood or adolescent antisocial behavior
V65.20 Malingering
V61.10 Marital problem

V15.81 Noncompliance with medical treatment
V62.20 Occupational problem
V61.20 Parent-child problem
V62.81 Other interpersonal problem
V61.80 Other specified family circumstances
V62.89 Phase of life problem or other life circumstance problem
V62.82 Uncomplicated bereavement

ADDITIONAL CODES

300.90 Unspecified mental disorder (nonpsychotic)
V71.09*No diagnosis or condition on Axis I

799.90*Diagnosis or condition deferred on Axis I
V71.09*No diagnosis or condition on Axis II
799.90*Diagnosis or condition deferred on Axis II

MULTIAXIAL SYSTEM

Axis I   Clinical Syndromes
          V Codes
Axis II   Developmental Disorders
          Personality Disorders
Axis III Physical Disorders and Conditions
Axis IV   Severity of Psychosocial Stressors
Axis V   Global Assessment of Functioning

From American Psychiatric Association: Diagnostic and Statistical Manual of Mental Disorders, 3rd Edition, Revised. Washington, DC, American Psychiatric Association, 1987. By permission of the publisher.

CODING AND DIAGNOSTIC DIFFERENCES BETWEEN DSM-III-R AND ICD-9-CM

The table below lists DSM-III-R codes that have fourth and fifth digit zeros not found in ICD-9-CM.

DSM-III-R Code	to	ICD-9-CM Code	DSM-III-R Code	to	ICD-9-CM Code
290.00		290.0	302.60		302.6
290.30		290.3	302.90		302.9
291.00		291.0	307.00		307.0
291.10		291.1	307.10		307.1
291.20		291.2	307.30		307.3
291.30		291.3	307.60		307.6
291.40		291.4	307.70		307.7
291.80		291.8	309.00		309.0

DSM-III-R Code	to	ICD-9-CM Code	DSM-III-R Code	to	ICD-9-CM Code
292.00		292.0	309.30		309.3
292.90		292.9	309.40		309.4
293.00		293.0	309.90		309.9
294.00		294.0	310.10		310.1
294.10		294.1	311.00		311
294.80		294.8	312.90		312.9
296.70		296.7	313.00		313.0
297.10		297.1	315.10		315.1
297.30		297.3	315.40		315.4
298.80		298.8	315.90		315.9
298.90		298.9	316.00		316
300.30		300.3	317.00		317
300.40		300.4	318.00		318.0
300.60		300.6	318.10		318.1
300.70		300.7	318.20		318.2
300.90		300.9	319.00		319
301.00		301.0	799.90		799.9
301.40		301.4	V61.10		V61.1
301.60		301.6	V61.80		V61.8
301.70		301.7	V62.20		V62.2
302.20		302.2	V62.30		V62.3
302.30		302.3	V65.20		V65.2
302.40		302.4			

Below are listed DSM-III-R diagnoses with different ICD-9-CM codes.

DSM-III-R	Diagnoses	ICD-9-CM
294.80	Organic mental disorder NOS	294.9
305.30	Hallucinogen hallucinosis	292.12
307.40	Parasomnia NOS	307.47
312.39	Impulse control disorder NOS	312.30
780.50	Hypersomnia related to known organic factor	780.54
780.50	Insomnia related to known organic factor	780.52
780.54	Primary hypersomnia	307.44
V40.00	Borderline intellectual functioning	V62.89

MENTAL RETARDATION (AXIS II DIAGNOSIS)

Degree of Severity	IQ
Mild	50–55 to approximately 70
Moderate	35–40 to 50–55
Severe	20–25 to 35–40
Profound	below 20 or 25

From American Psychiatric Association: Diagnostic and Statistical Manual of Mental Disorders, 3rd Edition, Revised. Washington, DC, American Psychiatric Association, 1987. By permission of the publisher.

SEVERITY OF PSYCHOSOCIAL STRESSORS SCALE (AXIS IV): ADULTS

		Examples of stressors	
Code	Term	Acute events	Enduring circumstances
1	None	No acute events that may be relevant to the disorder	No enduring circumstances that may be relevant to the disorder
2	Mild	Broke up with boyfriend or girlfriend; started or graduated from school; child left home	Family arguments; job dissatisfaction; residence in high-crime neighborhood
3	Moderate	Marriage; marital separation; loss of job; retirement; miscarriage	Marital discord; serious financial problems; trouble with boss; being a single parent
4	Severe	Divorce; birth of first child	Unemployment; poverty
5	Extreme	Death of spouse; serious physical illness diagnosed; victim of rape	Serious chronic illness in self or child; ongoing physical or sexual abuse
6	Catastrophic	Death of child; suicide of spouse; devastating natural disaster	Captivity as hostage; concentration camp experience

		Examples of stressors	
Code	Term	Acute events	Enduring circumstances
0	Inadequate information, or no change in condition		

SEVERITY OF PSYCHOSOCIAL STRESSORS SCALE (AXIS IV): CHILDREN AND ADOLESCENTS

		Examples of stressors	
Code	Term	Acute events	Enduring circumstances
1	None	No acute events that may be relevant to the disorder	No enduring circumstances that may be relevant to the disorder
2	Mild	Broke up with boyfriend or girlfriend; change of school	Overcrowded living quarters; family arguments
3	Moderate	Expelled from school; birth of sibling	Chronic disabling illness in parent; chronic parental discord
4	Severe	Divorce of parents; unwanted pregnancy; arrest	Harsh or rejecting parents; chronic life-threatening illness in parent; multiple foster home placements
5	Extreme	Sexual or physical abuse; death of a parent	Recurrent sexual or physical abuse
6	Catastrophic	Death of both parents	Chronic life-threatening illness
0	Inadequate information, or no change in condition		

From American Psychiatric Association: Diagnostic and Statistical Manual of Mental Disorders, 3rd Edition, Revised. Washington, DC, American Psychiatric Association, 1987. By permission of the publisher.

GLOBAL ASSESSMENT OF FUNCTIONING SCALE (GAF SCALE, AXIS V)

Consider psychological, social, and occupational functioning on a hypothetical continuum of mental health–illness. Do not include impairment in functioning due to physical (or environmental) limitations.

Note: Use intermediate codes when appropriate, e.g., 45, 68, 72.

Code

90 _____ Absent or minimal symptoms (e.g., mild anxiety before an exam), good functioning in all areas, interested and involved in a wide range of activities, socially effective, generally satisfied with life, no more than everyday problems or concerns (e.g., an occasional argument with family members).

81

80 _____ If symptoms are present, they are transient and expectable reactions to psychosocial stressors (e.g., difficulty concentrating after family argument); no more than slight impairment in social, occupational, or school functioning (e.g., temporarily falling behind in school work).

71

70 _____ Some mild symptoms (e.g., depressed mood and mild insomnia) OR some difficulty in social, occupational, or school functioning (e.g., occasional truancy, or theft within the household), but generally functioning pretty well, has some meaningful interpersonal relationships.

61

60 _____ Moderate symptoms (e.g., flat affect and circumstantial speech, occasional panic attacks) OR moderate difficulty in social, occupational, or school functioning (e.g., few friends, conflicts with co-workers).

51

50
— Serious symptoms (e.g., suicidal ideation, severe obsessional rituals, frequent shoplifting) OR any serious impairment in social, occupational, or school functioning (e.g., no friends, unable to keep a job).
41
—
40
— Some impairment in reality testing or communication (e.g., speech is at times illogical, obscure, or irrelevant) OR major impairment in several areas, such as work or school, family relations, judgment, thinking, or mood (e.g., depressed man avoids friends, neglects family, and is unable to work; child frequently beats up younger children, is defiant at home, and is failing at school).
31
—
30
— Behavior is considerably influenced by delusions or hallucinations OR serious impairment in communication or judgment (e.g., sometimes incoherent, acts grossly inappropriately, suicidal preoccupation) OR inability to function in almost all areas (e.g., stays in bed all day; no job, home, or friends).
21
—
20
— Some danger of hurting self or others (e.g., suicide attempts without clear expectation of death, frequently violent, manic excitement) OR occasionally fails to maintain minimal personal hygiene (e.g., smears feces) OR gross impairment in communication (e.g., largely incoherent or mute).
11
—
10
— Persistent danger of severely hurting self or others (e.g., recurrent violence) OR persistent inability to maintain minimal personal hygiene or serious suicidal act with clear expectation of death.
1
—
0
— Inadequate information.

THE HOLMES SOCIAL READJUSTMENT RATING SCALE

Note: Several scales for measuring severity of stressors are available. This well-known scale is included in this manual as a supplement to Axis IV of DSM-III-R. A total score of 300 or more points in 1 year has been correlated with increased incidence of physical illness.

Life Event	Mean Value
1. Death of spouse	100
2. Divorce	73
3. Marital separation from mate	65
4. Detention in jail or other institution	63
5. Death of a close family member	63
6. Major personal injury or illness	53
7. Marriage	50
8. Being fired at work	47
9. Marital reconciliation with mate	45
10. Retirement from work	45
11. Major change in the health or behavior of a family member	44
12. Pregnancy	40
13. Sexual difficulties	39
14. Gaining a new family member (through birth, adoption, oldster moving in, etc.)	39
15. Major business readjustment (merger, reorganization, bankruptcy, etc.)	39
16. Major change in financial state (a lot worse off or a lot better off than usual)	38
17. Death of a close friend	37
18. Changing to a different line of work	36
19. Major change in the number of arguments with spouse (either a lot more or a lot less than usual regarding child rearing, personal habits, etc.)	35
20. Taking on a mortgage greater than $10,000 (purchasing a home, business, etc.)	31
21. Foreclosure on a mortgage or loan	30
22. Major change in responsibilities at work (promotion, demotion, lateral transfer)	29
23. Son or daughter leaving home (marriage, attending college, etc.)	29
24. In-law troubles	29
25. Outstanding personal achievement	28
26. Wife beginning or ceasing work outside the home	26

Life Event	Mean Value
27. Beginning or ceasing formal schooling	26
28. Major change in living conditions (building a new home, remodeling, deterioration of home or neighborhood)	25
29. Revision of personal habits (dress, manners, associations, etc.)	24
30. Troubles with the boss	23
31. Major change in working hours or conditions	20
32. Change in residence	20
33. Changing to a new school	20
34. Major change in usual type or amount of recreation	19
35. Major change in church activities (a lot more or a lot less than usual)	19
36. Major change in social activities (clubs, dancing, movies, visiting, etc.)	18
37. Taking on a mortgage or loan less than $10,000 (purchasing a car, TV, freezer, etc.)	17
38. Major change in sleeping habits (a lot more or a lot less sleep or change in part of day when asleep)	16
39. Major change in number of family get-togethers (a lot more or a lot less than usual)	15
40. Major change in eating habits (a lot more or a lot less food intake or very different meal hours or surroundings)	15
41. Vacation	13
42. Christmas	12
43. Minor violations of the law (traffic tickets, jaywalking, disturbing the peace, etc.)	11

From Holmes TH: Life situations, emotions, and disease. Psychosomatics 19:747–754, 1978. By permission of The Academy of Psychosomatic Medicine.

SPECIALIZED INTERVIEWS AND ASSESSMENTS

ASSESSMENT OF POTENTIAL FOR VIOLENCE

This is notoriously difficult; however, points to consider include the following.

1. Patient's current mental status: quality of judgment, current state of arousal, any impairment of consciousness, evidence of psychosis
2. Degree of impulsivity as evidenced by past behaviors (e.g., driving violations, job history, pattern of spending money, social/sexual relationships, risk-taking behaviors)
3. Access to weapons, martial-arts training, military training, aggressive sports or hobbies
4. Use of intoxicating substances
5. Past history of violent activity and its circumstances; history of self-destructive activity; history of property destruction
6. Criminal record
7. Current medical or psychiatric disease; history of head injury, seizure
8. Predisposing personality traits or disorders (e.g., paranoid, antisocial, borderline)
9. Childhood exposure to violence, history of abuse (physical or sexual), or "chaotic" childhood with multiple or neglecting caretakers
10. Ability of patient to express frustration or anger by nonviolent means; consider verbal skills, intelligence, past coping mechanisms, current social-support network

Finally, does the patient have a specific target or plan for violent behavior? If so, consider means to protect patient or others. Document the evaluation and clinical judgment.

See also:

Reid WH, Balis GU: Evaluation of the violent patient. Psychiatr Update 6:491–509, 1987.

Lion JR, Reid WH (eds): Assaults Within Psychiatric Facilities. New York, Grune & Stratton, 1983.

Tardiff K (ed): The Violent Patient. Psychiatr Clin North Am 11:499–679, 1988.

MANAGEMENT OF VIOLENT PATIENTS IN THE EMERGENCY ROOM

The primary concern of the examining psychiatrist in this setting is the safety of the patient and other persons in the area (including oneself). Potentially violent patients can generally be approached with a calm, reassuring, and nonthreatening manner. Many agitated patients will become calm in the presence of an examiner who is calm and genuinely interested in understanding their experience.

Points to remember:

1. Have security personnel on standby until the situation is controlled, outside or even inside room.
2. Ascertain whether any weapons are present and remove them from the area if possible.
3. Sometimes the offer of a snack or cigarette can be calming.
4. Keep the environment quiet and simple.
5. Don't hurry.
6. Assess need for antipsychotic treatment or sedation. A neuroleptic or benzodiazepine, or both, can be given. Example: Haloperidol, 5-10 mg im or po, or lorazepam, 1-2 mg im or po; may be used separately or together.
7. Offer medication on a voluntary basis first. Involuntary administration of medication should be a last resort; some states and institutions require a restraining order for this.

    Restraining order: A temporary restraining order or "hold" order is placed when the patient is judged in imminent danger of hurting himself or herself or others and refuses appropriate treatment. This permits involuntary hospitalization but does not automatically justify the use of chemical or physical restraints. In some states security personnel may not restrain a patient unless a "hold" order has been signed by the responsible physician. See guidelines on the following pages.

    Transfer: When the patient is calm or adequately controlled, the patient may be transferred to an appropriate care setting. Notify the receiving unit of the patient's condition and transfer the patient with adequate personnel when the unit is prepared.

See also: Soloff PH: Emergency management of violent patients. Psychiatr Update 6:510–536, 1987.

Procedure for Instituting a Temporary Hold Order

1. Inform patient of your intent; inform patient's family and the physician of record.
2. In the presence of a witness, read to the patient the statement of patient's rights.
3. Give patient a copy of statement of patient's rights and place one copy in chart.
4. Fill out physician's statement regarding the need for temporary hold, with copies for patient and legal authorities as required.
5. In most states the hold period is 72 hours, excluding weekends and holidays.
6. Document steps 1–4 in chart, including the patient's response.

Guidelines for Seclusion and Restraints

Laws and policies vary greatly. These possible indications for seclusion or restraint are offered as guidelines.

1. To prevent imminent harm to the patient or other persons when less restrictive means of control are not effective or appropriate
2. To prevent serious disruption of the ward milieu or significant damage to the physical environment
3. As part of an ongoing treatment plan directed at specific problematic behaviors
4. To decrease the external stimulation a patient receives from the ward enviroment
5. In response to an appropriate request by the patient for seclusion or restraint, in accord with the indications listed above

Reasons for seclusion should be documented in the patient's chart and reviewed regularly. Patients in seclusion should be evaluated promptly and at frequent intervals as dictated by the patient's status. Time spent in seclusion or restraints should be minimized. Food, water, use of toilet facilities, and staff contact should be offered frequently and this should be documented in the patient record.

ASSESSMENT OF RISK OF SUICIDE

Most patients respond well to a tactful, straightforward approach, especially after some rapport has developed during the interview. For example:

"Have you ever been so discouraged (sad/down/frustrated) that you've thought about killing yourself or ending your life?"

If yes, continue to determine:
Current thoughts of suicide
Patient's plan or means of suicide
Previous episodes of suicidal thoughts
Previous suicide attempts or gestures
Alternative means of coping (e.g., run away, call for help)

If no, one may inquire:
"Most people have thought about suicide. How did you decide you wouldn't kill yourself?"

Points to consider in assessing suicide risk:
Access to weapons
Lethality of plan
Patient's impulsivity
History of risk-taking behavior
Drug or alcohol abuse
Family history of suicide

It is occasionally useful to distinguish among:
Death wish (e.g., "Sometimes I wish I would go to sleep and never wake up.")
Suicidal ideation
Suicide gesture without intent to die
Nonlethal self-destructive activity (e.g., cutting or burning skin)
Suicidal intent with plan
Suicide attempt

With children it is especially important to inquire as to the child's belief about the lethality of a plan or attempt. For example, one child may ingest four aspirin in the sincere belief that this is lethal; another child may ingest an entire bottle of medication as an expression of anger without intending to die.

RISK FACTORS FOR SUICIDE

Major psychiatric disorder, especially depression or schizophrenia

Male > female (females make more attempts)

Psychiatric hospitalization, dismissal from psychiatric hospital in past 6–12 months

Whites > blacks and other minorities

Elderly and adolescent > middle-aged in general population

    Among psychiatric patients, peak ages:

        Men 25–40 years

        Women 35–50 years

Alcoholism, other substance abuse

Widowed or divorced > single > married

Previous suicide attempt

Unemployed or retired

Serious physical illness

Recent loss (personal, financial, social)

Living alone

Possible warning signs of impending suicide

Verbal: Direct "I'm going to shoot myself."

          Indirect "You would be better off if I were dead."

          Morbid preoccupation with death or suicide

Behavioral: Depressive syndrome

             Getting life in order

             Giving away possessions

             Failing grades, poor work performance

             Substance abuse

             Risk taking

             "Accidents" (may be disguised suicide attempts)

McAlpine DE: Suicide: recognition and management. Mayo Clin Proc 62:778–781, 1987.

Mann JJ, Stanley M: Suicide. Rev Psychiatry 7:287–426, 1988.

Clayton PJ: Suicide. Psychiatr Clin North Am 8:203–214, 1985.

CHEMICAL DEPENDENCY INTERVIEW

SPECIAL FEATURES OF THE CHEMICAL DEPENDENCY INTERVIEW

Points to include regarding drug use:
    Drug of choice
    Date and time of most recent use
    Amount and route of most recent use
    Habitual pattern and circumstances of use
    First exposure
    Source

Consequences of use
    Inquire as to:
        Health   Legal problems
        Family relationships   Education and career
        Social relationships   Religious status
        Finances   Psychological status

Previous attempts to cut down or control use and results

Previous treatment experience

Family history of substance use or abuse

SCREENING INTERVIEW FOR DIAGNOSIS OF ALCOHOLISM

Ask: 1. Do you drink?
        If no, ask:
     2. Could you tell me why? (looking for the abstaining alcoholic)
        If yes, ask:
     2. How do you drink? (looking for alcoholic patterns)
     3. Have you or close family members ever been concerned about your drinking?
     4. Has drinking ever caused problems in your life?

From Morse RM, Hurt RD: Screening for alcoholism. JAMA 242:2688–2690, 1979. By permission of Mayo Foundation.

SYMPTOMS SUGGESTIVE OF PROBLEM DRINKING

Preoccupation with drinking
Impulsive drinking
Gulping drinks
Inappropriate circumstances
Medicinal drinking
Solitary drinking
Secret drinking
Guilt after drinking
Hidden bottle or supply
Periodic attempts at abstinence
Social isolation

Missing appointments in order to drink
Daily use
Tolerance
Loss of control
DWI (driving while intoxicated) arrests
Personality change
Blackouts
Withdrawal symptoms
Morning drinking
Morning tremor

See also:

Manual on Alcoholism, 3rd Edition. Chicago, IL, American Medical Association, 1977.

Meyer RE: Alcoholism. Rev Psychiatry 8:265–380, 1989.

FORENSIC PSYCHIATRY

The forensic evaluation contains specialized elements and has a different emphasis than the clinical psychiatric evaluation. Patients should be advised of the purpose of the interview and that the usual doctor-patient relationship and confidentiality standards do not apply.

The following lists are included as reminders. State statutes vary. In any given case, psychiatrists are advised to consult with an attorney or court representative regarding local legislation and to clarify their involvement in the case.

Sources for this section and recommended reading include:

1. Gutheil TG, Appelbaum PS: Clinical Handbook of Psychiatry and the Law. New York, McGraw-Hill, 1982
2. Simon RI: Concise Guide to Clinical Psychiatry and the Law. Washington, DC, American Psychiatric Press, 1988
3. Stone AA: Legal issues, in Psychiatric Reference Book, 2nd Edition. Edited by Stern M. New York, Co Medica, 1985, pp 100–103; 112

CONFIDENTIALITY

In a therapeutic relationship the patient "owns" the information revealed to the physician and therefore controls its distribution. (The patient record is the property of the physician, although most states allow the patient access to the record.) Patient confidentiality should be breached without consent only to protect the patient or another person from imminent grave harm, or when mandated by law (as in reporting child abuse). Many situations that seem to require disclosure of privileged information can be legally and ethically approached by including the patient in the decision of what information will be disclosed. For example, a minor can be enlisted to discuss treatment progress with parents, or a legal report can be discussed with the patient prior to release to an attorney.

Written authorization for release of information should be obtained for each disclosure and kept in the permanent record. The obligation of confidentiality remains in the event of the patient's death.

ELEMENTS OF INFORMED CONSENT

A. The patient must have *information about* the treatment under consideration.
   1. Description of the treatment
   2. Reasons for the treatment (discussion of illness or problem)
   3. Potential benefits from this treatment versus benefits from other treatments, including no treatment
   4. Potential risks, including common risks and rare but potentially serious risks such as death; include risks of alternative treatments and of no treatment
   5. Right to withdraw from treatment at any time
B. The patient must give *voluntary* (without coercion) consent.
C. The patient must have *capacity to consent*.
   1. Age of majority
   2. Of "sound mind"—able to understand and reason about the decision
   3. Be able to communicate the choice
D. The physician should document this discussion and the patient's decision (consent or refusal) regarding the treatment options. The capacity of the patient to give consent and the voluntary nature of the consent should be noted.

E. Because many patients do not recall all information presented, written materials or videotapes are a useful adjunct, and their use may also be noted in the chart.

F. Special consideration must be given to cases in which the patient is unable to give informed consent (e.g., children or mentally incompetent patients). A legally responsible guardian may consent for the patient. When a responsible family member is unavailable or the identity of the guardian is not clear, a court-appointed guardian may be required.

INVOLUNTARY COMMITMENT

All states permit brief (72 hours) emergency hospitalization without the patient's consent if the patient is judged by a responsible physician to be mentally ill and a danger to self or others, or unable to care for his or her own basic needs. For continued hospitalization, civil commitment proceedings must take place, beginning with a "probable cause" hearing. Commitment proceedings vary but usually involve demonstration of risk of dangerousness to self or others of such magnitude as to warrant removal of the patient's civil liberties by involuntary hospitalization. Some states provide for civil commitment of severely mentally ill persons without demonstration of dangerousness. Standards and procedures for long-term commitment vary. Involuntary treatment administered to committed persons is a separate and controversial legal issue; regional standards apply.

COMPETENCY TO MAKE A WILL (TESTAMENTARY CAPACITY)

Individual must understand:
1. Nature and extent of his or her property
2. Natural objects of his or her bounty (identity and relationship of usual beneficiaries)
3. Nature and effect of making a will

COMPETENCY TO STAND TRIAL

The defendant must be able to participate in his or her own defense. To this end, the individual must:
1. Understand the nature of the proceedings
2. Be able to communicate and cooperate with his or her attorney

CRIMINAL RESPONSIBILITY (INSANITY DEFENSE)

This area of law is currently controversial and under active study. The American Law Institute Test is now widely accepted. It states that a defendant may be found "not guilty by reason of insanity" if: 1) because of mental disease or defect (excluding antisocial conduct disorders), 2) a person lacks the capacity to *appreciate* the criminality of his or her conduct, and/or 3) is unable to *conform* his or her behavior to the requirements of the law.

The relevant determination for psychiatrists is the defendant's mental status at the time of the alleged crime.

In some states a defendant may be found "guilty but mentally ill" and sentenced accordingly.

MALPRACTICE

Malpractice is a tort (civil suit) that involves a demonstration of physician negligence to provide "reasonable care." The level of proof required is a "preponderance of the evidence" (about 75% certainty). The four elements of malpractice include: 1) demonstration of physician *duty* to care for the patient, 2) *negligent* practice has occurred, 3) the patient has sustained some *harm*, and 4) the harm was *caused* by physician negligence. This formula is summarized as "the four Ds"; the *duty* to care exists, and *deviation* from the usual standard of care has resulted in *damage* to the patient that resulted *directly* from the deviant care. Psychiatrists are advised to:

1. Follow good ethical practice (outlined in the AMA guidelines, with annotations for psychiatry published by the APA), with primary concern for the patient's welfare.
2. Obtain informed consent for treatment and procedures.
3. Maintain legible clinical records, and document treatment discussions, phone calls, risk-benefit judgments, recommendations, and instructions given to patients and families.
4. Obtain physical and laboratory examinations prior to prescribing somatic therapies.
5. Document transfer of care or termination of care decisions and the provisions for the patient to receive ongoing care.

DUTY TO WARN

The duty to warn third parties who may be endangered by the actions of a patient is a logical extension of the physician's obligation to "do no harm." Failure to intervene constitutes negligence if a patient is judged to pose a serious threat to an identified person. However, warning a third party can potentially destroy the therapeutic relationship and may unduly frighten the person warned. The physician is advised to:

1. Carefully assess the potential for violence and the seriousness and likelihood of the threat.
2. Consider any means by which the potential for violence may be reduced (e.g., hospitalization, medication, intensified treatment, disposal of weapons).
3. Enlist the patient's cooperation or consent in warning a third party if possible.
4. In warning a third party, limit disclosure of information to that required for clarity.
5. Document the risk-benefit judgment and the actions taken.
6. Notify law enforcement.

PSYCHIATRIC ASSESSMENT OF A CHILD

SUGGESTED INTERVIEW FORMAT

This outline offers key elements to be included in a child psychiatry assessment.

   I. Overview
      A. Establish rapport
         1. Meet the child and accompanying adults
         2. Find out why the child thinks he or she is being seen
         3. Discuss the nature and procedure of the interview
         4. Explain that information given is confidential with the exception of protecting the child and others from imminent harm

B. Gather general information
  1. Chief complaint from child and from adult
  2. Identifying information
     a. Age, school grade, physical condition, intelligence
     b. Character, temperament, judgment, attitudes
  3. History of present illness

II. Developmental history
A. Family
  1. Structure of evaluation should include individual interviews with the parents
  2. Note child's attitude toward each parent
  3. Child's relationships with siblings
  4. Family psychiatric history
  5. History of parents' own childhoods
     a. Relationships with their parents and siblings
     b. Discipline methods used; evidence of abuse or dysfunction
     c. Level of education and current occupation
  6. Circumstances of patient's birth; if adopted, circumstances and motivation for adoption
B. Developmental milestones
  1. Physical
     a. Pregnancy, delivery, feeding, and weaning; neonatal illnesses
     b. Early or significant medical illness or injury
     c. Neuromuscular development of speech, motor milestones (sit, stand, walk, first words, play)
  2. Behavioral
     a. Toilet training and other training—response to discipline, methods used
     b. Reactions to beginning day care or school
     c. Sleep patterns; sleep disturbances
     d. Phobias
     e. Habit disorders (e.g., bed-wetting and thumb-sucking)
C. Significant events: move, parent's death, divorce

    D. Current level of functioning
       1. School performance
       2. Hobbies and extracurricular activities
       3. Peer relationships
       4. Relationships with adults other than parents
       5. Unusual habits or habit disorders
       6. Aims and ambitions
       7. Current health and medications

III. Interview with the child—possible topics of discussion:

    A. Child's ideas about the problem
       1. Expectation for outcome
       2. What child would like to change in self or others
       3. "What problems have we not talked about yet?"
    B. Symptom review
       1. Vegetative symptoms
       2. Anxiety symptoms
       3. Psychotic symptoms
       4. Suicidal ideation, other self-destructive acts
       5. Ruminations or acts of violence
       6. Substance use
       7. Victimization experiences
    C. Mental status examination
       1. Orientation, memory, communication skills
       2. Cognitive mental state—include estimate of intelligence and academic skills
       3. Mood and affect
       4. Drawings—house/tree/person, self-portrait, kinetic family drawing

IV. Consider other information to be sought

    A. Psychological testing
    B. Medical consultations—pediatric, neurologic
    C. School records, interview with teachers
    D. Interviews with other significant adults (noncustodial parents, grandparent, social worker)
    E. Previous treatment or evaluation records

MENTAL STATUS EXAMINATION OF A CHILD

This is a useful format for organizing the report of the pediatric mental status examination.

1. Appearance
2. Mood or affect
3. Orientation and perception
4. Coping mechanisms
   a. Major defenses
   b. Expression and control of affectional and aggressive impulses
5. Neuromuscular integration
6. Thought processes and verbalization; speech quality; vocabulary
7. Fantasy
   a. Dreams
   b. Drawings
   c. Wishes
   d. Play
8. Superego
   a. Ego ideals and values
   b. Integration into personality
9. Concept of self
   a. Object relations
   b. Identification
10. Awareness of problems
11. Estimate of intelligence
12. Summary of Mental Status Examination

From Simmons JE: Psychiatric Examination of Children, 4th Edition. Philadelphia, PA, Lea & Febiger, 1987. By permission of the publisher.

THE HOSPITAL CONSULTATION INTERVIEW

The evaluation of a patient in the hospital consultation setting has some special considerations in addition to calling for good history-taking and interviewing skills. The clinician should understand the consultation request as a call for assistance by the primary physician, and in most cases, the evaluation should proceed quickly. Liaison psychiatry is an associated but separate field, as when a psychiatrist or psychiatric team is permanently affiliated with a medical service.

I. **Elements of the hospital consultation**
   A. Be of service to the consulting physician
      1. Understand the nature of the consultation. If the referral is vague, contact the referring physician to learn the reason for the referral and the desired assistance. It is helpful to know how the patient has been prepared for the consultation.
      2. Answer the question. Unrelated psychiatric issues may surface during the evaluation. These should be brought to the attention of the referring service, but not to the exclusion of the original request.
      3. In composing the consultation note, strive to be complete, brief, and direct. Avoid technical jargon.
   B. Be of service to the patient
      1. As with any patient evaluation, gather background and collateral information. Hospital patients often have accompanying relatives who may give valuable information. Nurses' observations of behavior should be noted.
      2. Offer a clear diagnostic and management plan to the referring physician and the patient. If the limitations of the setting do not permit a definitive diagnosis, briefly explain the nature of the limitations and state the differential diagnosis along with the management plan.

3. Follow the patient's progress during the hospital stay. If requested or where appropriate, assist in making arrangements for outpatient follow-up.

II. Common reasons to seek psychiatric consultation
A. Diagnosis of suspected psychiatric illness
B. Assistance in management of psychiatric disorder; transfer to psychiatric service
C. Substance abuse disorder
D. Somatization disorder
E. Psychosocial factors exacerbating physical condition
F. Noncompliance or refusal of essential treatment
G. Staff-patient conflicts
H. Supportive treatment of patient or family during catastrophic illness
I. Ethical conflicts

III. Elements to include in the consultation evaluation
The emphasis of the hospital consultation evaluation will vary according to the nature of the problem and the specific referral request. However, all consultation evaluations should include the basic elements of the general psychiatric evaluation with particular attention to the following.
A. History of present illness, including the current medical record, results of examinations and tests, and response to treatment
B. Past medical history
C. Past psychiatric history
D. Current medicines
E. Substance use
F. Developmental and social history
G. Family medical and psychiatric history
H. Current mental status examination

NARCOTIC ANALGESICS (ORAL AND PARENTERAL) FOR SEVERE PAIN

The consulting psychiatrist is sometimes asked to evaluate patients who require management of acute severe pain. This table describes narcotics used for control of acute pain.

	Route*	Equianalgesic dose (mg)†	Duration (h)	Plasma half-life (h)	Comments
Narcotic agonists					
Morphine	im	10	4–6	2–3.5	Standard for comparison; also available in slow-release tablets
	po	60	4–7		
Codeine	im	130	4–6	3	Biotransformed to morphine; useful as initial narcotic analgesic
	po	60	4–6		
Oxycodone	im	15	3–5	...	Short acting; available alone or as 5-mg dose in combination with aspirin and acetaminophen
	po	30			
Levorphanol (Levo–Dromoran)	im	2	4–6	12–16	Good oral potency, requires careful titration in initial dosing because of drug accumulation
	po	4	4–7		
Hydromorphone (Dilaudid)	im	1.5	4–5	2–3	Available in high-potency injectable form (10 mg/ml) for cachectic patients and as rectal suppositories; more soluble than morphine
	po	7.5	4–6		
Oxymorphone (Numorphan)	im	1	4–6	2–3	Available in parenteral and rectal-suppository forms only
	pr	10	4–6		
Meperidine (Demerol)	im	75	3–4	3–4 (Normeperidine)	Contraindicated in patients with renal disease or those taking monoamine oxidase inhibitors; accumulation of active toxic metabolite normeperidine produces central nervous system excitation
	po	300	4–6	12–16	

Drug	Route	Dose	Duration	Half-life	Comments
Methadone (Dolophine)	im po	10 20		15–30	Good oral potency; requires careful titration of the initial dose to avoid drug accumulation
Mixed agonist-antagonist drugs					
Pentazocine (Talwin)	im po	60 180	4–6 4–7	2–3	Limited use for cancer pain; psychotomimetic effects with dose escalation; available only in combination with naloxone, aspirin, or acetaminophen; may precipitate withdrawal in patients physically dependent on opiates
Nalbuphine (Nubain)	im	10	4–6	5	Not available orally; less severe psychotomimetic effects than pentazocine; may precipitate withdrawal in patients physically dependent on opiates
Butorphanol (Stadol)	im	2	4–6	2.5–3.5	Not available orally; produces psychotomimetic effects; may precipitate withdrawal in patients physically dependent on opiates
Partial agonists					
Buprenorphine (Temgesic)	im sl	0.4 0.8	4–6 5–6	?	No psychotomimetic effects; may precipitate withdrawal in tolerant patients

*im, intramuscular; po, oral; pr, rectal; sl, sublingual.

†Based on single-dose studies in which an intramuscular dose of each drug listed was compared with morphine to establish the relative potency. Oral doses are those recommended when changing from a parenteral to an oral route. For patients without prior narcotic exposure, the recommended oral starting dose is 30 mg for morphine, 5 mg for methadone, 2 mg for levorphanol, and 4 mg for hydromorphone.

From Foley KM: The treatment of cancer pain. N Engl J Med 313:84–95, 1985. By permission of the journal.

PSYCHOLOGY REFERRALS: CONSULTATION AND ASSESSMENT

I. The Referral Process

A clearly worded referral request is essential to gain the most benefit from a psychological consultation. A telephone call or personal conversation is preferred by many psychologists, but a written statement will suffice if it is legible and well formulated.

A. Completing the Consultation Request
   1. Ask an explicit question. For example, "Will relaxation therapy help patient cope with anxiety?"
   2. If the reason for referral is more general, briefly describe the nature of the problem. For example, "Question of dementia of Alzheimer's type; need baseline assessment of cognitive and memory functions."

B. Examples of Poor Referrals
   1. No referring document or question.
   2. "Psychometrics"—Insufficient information will require a call to the referring physician and delay the assessment.
   3. "Elective mute. Obtain verbal IQ."—If patient is unable to cooperate with standard interview and testing procedure, direct consultation with the psychologist is advised.

II. Psychological Consultations and Assessments

Although often asked to incorporate information from psychological test batteries into patient evaluations, few psychiatrists receive detailed training in this area. The choice of a specific test in a particular clinical setting depends on the nature of the clinical problem, the type of information sought, the degree of accuracy required, and the training and preference of the examiner.

What follows are examples of frequently used psychological instruments, arranged by the type of assessment in which each is used. Both detailed instruments and screening tests are listed here, provided they are in common use. This section is organized as follows.

A. Personality and Psychopathology Assessment

B. Behavioral Assessment

C. Cognitive and Developmental Assessment

D. Academic Assessment

E. Neuropsychological Evaluation

F. Occupational Interest and Aptitude Evaluation

For each test the following information is presented: name of the instrument (abbreviation), age range for which it is appropriate, time needed to complete the test, and other comments.

A. Personality and Psychopathology Assessment
   Formal testing procedures are a useful adjunct to the clinical interview in understanding the nature of a patient's personality or psychopathology.
   1. Objective instruments for personality traits and psychopathology.
      a. Minnesota Multiphasic Personality Inventory (MMPI)*
         Adult and adolescent norms available. Self-administered. 45–90 minutes, 566 items. Scored on 10 clinical and 4 validity scales; numerous research and supplemental scales available. See description of scales following this section.
      b. Symptom Checklist 90—Revised (SCL-90-R)
         16 years and older. Self-administered. 12–15 minutes, 90 items. Scored on 3 global indices of psychic distress and 9 symptom dimensions.
      c. Millon Clinical Multiaxial Inventory (MCMI); Millon Adolescent Personality Inventory
         Adults; adolescent form available. Self-administered. 25 minutes, 175 items. Scored on 20 clinical scales and 2 correction scales, using DSM-III terminology.
      d. Sixteen Personality Factor Questionnaire (16PF)
         16 years and older. Self-administered. 45–60 minutes, 374 items. Not a measure of psychopathology. Scored on 24 scales with 16 primary factor scales of personality traits.

---

*Further information is presented later in this book.

2. Projective instruments to measure personality traits and areas of major psychic conflict.

The validity and reliability of projective tests have been disputed when applied to children and adolescents. Nevertheless, the tests are widely used and helpful when properly interpreted.

a. Rorschach

Children, adolescents, adults. Trained examiner displays 10 pictures of achromatic or colored inkblots; patient's verbal responses are recorded and scored. 60–90 minutes. The Exner system is a widely accepted method of scoring.

b. Thematic Apperception Test (TAT)

Children, adolescents, adults. Trained examiner displays cards illustrating family and social situations. Patient tells a story about each scene. 60–90 minutes.

c. Sentence Completion Test

Children, adolescents, adults. Many variations of this test are available. Self-administered. 15–30 minutes. Patient completes sentence fragments.

d. Draw A Person

Children, adolescents, adults. Several forms of this test and scoring methods are available. 5–20 minutes. Patient is asked to "draw a person" on a blank page. Scoring may reflect cognitive functioning as well as projective elements.

B. Behavioral Assessment

Behavioral medicine involves understanding stimulus-response cycles that lead to patterns of problematic behavior. Assessment involves various instruments, including self-report inventories, observational checklists, and physiologic responses. These must be valid and reliable instruments for measuring the target behavior.

1. Examples of self-report inventories.

a. Beck Depression Inventory

Adults. Self-administered. 15–20 minutes, 21 multiple-choice items. Scored as an index of severity of depressed mood, with a list of major symptoms.

b. Self-Administered Alcoholism Screening Test (SAAST)

Adults. Self-administered. 10 minutes, 37 items patterned after the Michigan Alcoholism Screening Test interview. A spouse observation checklist is available.

2. Examples of observation checklists.
    a. Conners Parent-Teacher Rating Scale

    Children, adolescents. Self-administered forms for parents and teachers. 10 minutes. Child is rated 0–3 on several items that describe immature, hyperactive, somatic, or aggressive behaviors.
    b. Child Behavior Checklist (Achenbach)

    4–18 years. Rating scales completed by parent, teacher, or observer; a self-report form is available for youths 11–18 years old. Scores are obtained for social competence (activities, social, school) and manifest behavior problems (internalizing, externalizing) and several factor scales (e.g., hyperactivity).
    c. Personality Inventory for Children—Revised (PIC)

    3–16 years. Rating scale completed by parent. 600 items similar to MMPI. Yields 3 validity and 12 clinical scales; 17 research scales can also be scored.
3. Physiologic measures.

    Many organic disorders are caused or exacerbated by physiologic arousal involving the skeletal muscles and autonomic nervous system. Assessment may include electronic measurement of peripheral skin temperature, electrodermal conductance, pulse rate, or muscle tension. Physiologic measures of stress are tailored to the age of the patient and the nature of the chief complaint. Typically these measurements are incorporated into a biofeedback treatment program to help patients develop self-regulatory skills for these processes. An example would be the use of EMG and skin temperature recordings to augment relaxation training in the treatment of tension headache and cervical pain.

C. Cognitive and Developmental Assessment

General screening of cognitive abilities usually requires 2 or more hours for the administration of intelligence, learning, and memory tests.

1. Intelligence testing.
    a. Wechsler Adult Intelligence Scale–Revised (WAIS-R)*

    16 years and older. Trained examiner administers verbal and nonverbal tasks of problem-solving ability. 60–90 minutes, 11 subtests. Scoring: 11 subtest scores are

---

*Further information is presented later in this book.

grouped as Verbal and Performance IQ measures. These are combined to yield a Full Scale IQ.

b. Wechsler Intelligence Scale for Children (WISC-R)*

6–16 years. 50–75 minutes, 12 subtests yield Verbal, Performance, and Full Scale IQ scores.

c. Wechsler Preschool and Primary Scale of Intelligence (WPPSI)*

4–6.5 years. 60 minutes, 10 subtests yield Verbal, Performance, and Full Scale IQ scores.

d. Stanford-Binet Intelligence Scale

2 years to adult. Trained examiner administers multiple subtests of verbal and nonverbal abilities. 45–90 minutes, 15 subtests. Flexibility of subtest items makes this test preferred for some situations (e.g., developmental delay) in which the cognitive ability of the subject may vary unpredictably from clinical estimate.

e. Shipley Institute of Living Scale

15 years and older. Self-administered. 20 minutes, vocabulary and logical sequencing test may be used as a rapid estimate of intelligence.

2. Developmental assessment.

The psychologist is often confronted with patients requiring developmental assessment. When working with preschool children this involves a combination of verbal and performance tasks and observations from parents or caretakers.

a. Bayley Scales of Infant Development (BSID)

2–30 months. Trained examiner rates infant or toddler responses to various verbal and nonverbal stimuli. 45 minutes. Yields separate motor and mental development indices.

b. Cattell Infant Intelligence Scale

3–30 months. Trained examiner rates infant or toddler behaviors and verbalizations in response to various stimuli. 20–30 minutes. Scored as intelligence measure; some items overlap with Stanford-Binet.

c. Gesell Preschool Test

2.5–6 years. Trained examiner administers multiple verbal and nonverbal tasks. 40 minutes, 13 subtests.

---

*Further information is presented later in this book.

d. Denver Developmental Screening Test (DDST)

2 weeks to 6 years. Easily administered motor and language tasks supplemented with information from parent or caregiver. 15–20 minutes. Yields scores on four developmental scales: gross motor, fine motor–adaptive, language, personal-social.

3. Parent observation forms for developmental assessment.

a. Minnesota Child Development Inventory (MCDI)

1–6 years. Behavior checklist completed by primary parent or caregiver. 20–30 minutes, 320 items. Eight scales: general development, gross motor, fine motor, expressive language, comprehensive-conceptual (receptive language), situation-comprehensive, self-help, personal-social.

b. Kent Infant Development (KID) Scale

2–13 months. Rating scale completed by parent or caregiver. 30–40 minutes, 252 items. Six scales: cognitive, motor, social, language, self-help, and a summary score that may be used as a global estimate of development.

4. Structured interviews to assess development.

a. Vineland Adaptive Behavior Scales (VABS)

0–18 years and older if developmentally delayed. Structured interview. 20–60 minutes. Thirteen scores in areas of communication, daily living, socialization, motor skills, adaptive behavior, and maladaptive behavior.

b. Scales of Independent Behavior (SIB)

Infant to adult. Structured interview. 45–50 minutes. Yields information about adaptive behavior, expected range of independence, communication skills, self-care abilities, and instructional capabilities that may be combined with cognitive measures.

D. Academic Assessment

These tests focus on academic skills acquired in reading, spelling, or written language, calculation, and reasoning during elementary, junior, or senior high school. This type of assessment is useful to determine the presence or absence of a learning disability or in cases of unexplained deteriorating school performance.

1. Wide Range Achievement Test—Revised (WRAT-R)

5 years to adult. Trained examiner administers three aca-

demic tasks. 20–30 minutes. Measures word recognition, spelling from dictation, and calculation.

2. Woodcock-Johnson Psycho-Educational Battery (WJPEB)

3–80 years. Trained examiner. 90–120 minutes, 27 subtests. Yields 31 scores divided into three parts: cognitive ability, achievement, and interest. Subtests measure academic aptitude, reading skills (phonics, word recognition, comprehension), math-computation (calculation, application), and written language (spelling, proofreading) as well as academic areas of special interest.

3. Peabody Individual Achievement Test (PIAT)

Grades K to 12. Trained examiner. 30–40 minutes. Six scores: arithmetic, calculation, word recognition, reading comprehension, spelling, and general information.

4. Gray Oral Reading Test—Revised (GORT-R)

7–17 years. Screening task for reading fluency. 20–30 minutes. Standard scores and percentile ranks for oral reading rate, accuracy, and comprehension.

E. Neuropsychological Evaluation

Three or 4 hours may be needed for evaluation of the patient's ability to perform complex cognitive, memory, and sensory-perceptive tasks. Abilities measured may include speech reception and production, reasoning, alertness, concentration, memory function, learning ability, perceptual ability, information processing, cognitive flexibility, and fine motor skills. These measures are correlated with the integrity or dysfunction of the central nervous system. Because emotional factors such as depression or anxiety may interfere with the response quality, personality and psychopathology assessments may be required as part of the evaluation.

1. Halstead-Reitan Neuropsychological Test Battery

Child, adolescent, adult. Trained examiner administers a comprehensive battery of verbal and nonverbal tasks. Complete battery may take 4–6 hours. Examination of subtest performance gives detailed information as to neuropsychiatric functioning.

2. Luria-Nebraska Neuropsychological Battery

15 years and older. Trained examiner administers comprehensive battery of verbal and nonverbal tasks. 90–120 minutes, 269 items. Yields a profile of 16 scales.

3. Wechsler Memory Scale I, II—Revised (WMS-R)

Adolescent to adult. 60–90 minutes. Yields measures of immediate and delayed verbal and visual learning efficiency and memory functioning.

4. Bender Visual Motor Gestalt Test

5 years and older. Examiner displays 9 cards with geometric figures that patient copies. 10 minutes.

F. Occupational Interest and Aptitude Evaluation

This type of evaluation may be requested by the clinician as part of a rehabilitation, socialization, or after-care program to assist in educational or vocational planning.

1. Strong-Campbell Interest Inventory (SCII)

16 years and older. Self-administered. 20–40 minutes, 325 items. Computer scoring required. Yields scores of 6 general occupational themes, 23 basic interest scales, and 162 occupational scales.

2. Career Assessment Inventories (CAI)

Grade 8 through adult. Self-administered. 20–35 minutes, 305 items. Six general occupational themes, 22 occupational interest scales, and 91 occupational scales.

3. General Aptitude Test Battery (GATB)

16 years and older. Trained examiner administers 12 subtests covering 9 vocational aptitudes. 4 hours. The scores are related to the Comprehensive Directory of Occupational Titles prepared by the federal government.

III. Treatment Consultation

The primary goal of the behavioral treatment consultation is to arrange a management program that will decrease the frequency of unwanted behavior and increase the frequency of desired behavior. "Skill deficits" are assessed and a treatment plan is formulated which may include techniques such as systematic desensitization, flooding, modeling, progressive muscle relaxation, biofeedback, contingency management, reinforcement, time-out procedures, or cognitive behavioral therapies. Such approaches have been applied to a wide range of problems, including compulsive behaviors, stress management, childhood noncompliance, chronic pain, social skill deficits, sexual dysfunction, anxiety, and depressive disorders.

DESCRIPTION OF MMPI VALIDITY AND CLINICAL SCALES

Cannot Say (Q/?)

This validity index is not a scale in the usual sense of the term but simply represents the total number of items that have not been answered by the subject, including those marked both true and false. A high score suggests the subject may have been hesitant or uncomfortable with the ambiguity of many of the items and thus felt unable to respond, or it may simply represent an index of refusal to complete the task for other reasons.

Scale L (L)

An elevated score on the 15 items composing scale L suggests an effort, usually a conscious one, to create an impression of being a very "good" person in the sense of having high moral, social, and ethical values.

Scale F (F)

As the score on the 64 F items increases, the greater is the likelihood some factor has operated to invalidate the results. This might include poor reading comprehension or general reading ability, mental confusion, a deliberate desire to fake psychiatric disturbance, random marking of responses, or an error in scoring.

Scale K (K)

This 30-item scale measures a more subtle type of psychologic defensiveness than scale L. A moderate elevation indicates a view of the self as being well adjusted, capable, and confident. A very high elevation suggests an extremely positive degree of social and emotional well-being which is likely to be a denial of the patient's actual status. A portion of the K scale is added to five other scales (1,4,7,8,9) to improve clinical sensitivity (K correction).

Scale 1 (Hs; Hypochondriasis)

An elevation on scale 1 (33 items) suggests an undue concern with the state of one's body and possible preoccupation with symptoms of physical illness. In addition, high scorers are often typified by a sour or pessimistic view of life.

Scale 2 (D; Depression)

An elevation on scale 2 (60 items) indicates feelings of depression, sadness, pessimism, guilt, and passivity and a tendency to give up hope easily.

Scale 3 (Hy; Hysteria)

Scale 3 (60 items) seems to represent a continuum of psychologic maturity, with an elevated score characterizing people who tend to be self-centered, demanding, and superficial in their relationships with others and who use denial to such a degree that they might be appropriately described as wearing "rose-colored glasses."

Scale 4 ((Pd; Psychopathic deviate)

At moderate levels, scale 4 (50 items) describes interpersonal assertiveness and a desire for nonconformity, whereas marked elevations usually typify feelings of angry rebelliousness and a lack of identification with conventional social mores.

Scale 5 (Mf; Masculine-feminine)

Scale 5 (60 items) provides an index of the range of interests held by the individual and, for both sexes, the degree to which the subject identifies with traditional male or female roles.

Scale 6 (Pa; Paranoia)

Interpretation of elevations on scale 6 (40 items) can range from interpersonal sensitivity or oversensitivity to irritability or negative speculation about the possible motives or behavior of others and finally to the suspicious style of thinking that characterizes persons who have a paranoid type of personality.

Scale 7 (Pt; Psychasthenia)

An elevation on scale 7 (48 items) indicates generalized feelings of anxiety and discomfort. There is often excessive rumination about personal inadequacies, either real or imagined.

Scale 8 (Sc; Schizophrenia)

This scale is the longest (78 items) of those making up the basic MMPI profile and may be viewed as an index of comfort (or lack thereof) in interpersonal relationships. Elevations are associated with feelings of alienation or social detachment, which may extend to frank mental confusion or interpersonal aversiveness.

Scale 9 (Ma; Hypomania)

Scale 9 (46 items) assesses the subject's level of psychologic energy, with moderate elevations being characterized by talkativeness, distractibility, and physical restlessness and higher elevations being associated with impulsivity, impatience, irritability, or rapid mood swings.

Scale 0 (Si; Social introversion)

An elevation of this scale (70 items) indicates social introversion and a lack of desire to be with others; persons scoring low tend to enjoy social interactions and actively seek such contacts.

From Colligan RC, Osborne D, Swenson WM, et al: The aging MMPI: development of contemporary norms. Mayo Clin Proc 59:377–390, 1984. By permission of Mayo Foundation.

See also: Graham JR: The MMPI: A Practical Guide, 2nd Edition. New York, Oxford University Press, 1987.

DESCRIPTION OF WECHSLER SUBTESTS

The WAIS-R, WISC-R, and WPPSI are composed of similar subtests. Items on the WISC-R and WPPSI are simpler than those on the WAIS-R. The following is a list of the subtests with a brief explanation of each. They are presented in the order in which they are administered in the WAIS-R. Note that the subtests alternate between verbal and performance tasks.

1. *Information*—Several questions of general knowledge in multiple subject areas. Questions are designed to cover widely known subjects rather than academic areas.
2. *Picture Completion*—The patient must identify the missing element from each of multiple picture cards.
3. *Digit Span*—The patient repeats a sequence of digits after the examiner. Both forward and reverse recall are tested. (Not used in the WPPSI.)
4. *Picture Arrangement*—A set of picture cards must be arranged in sequence to tell a story. The end result resembles a cartoon panel. (Not used in the WPPSI.)

5. *Vocabulary*—The patient is asked to define a series of words of increasing difficulty. Words are presented orally and visually.

6. *Block Design*—The patient rearranges a cluster of red and white cubes to reproduce designs portrayed by the examiner's blocks or cards with printed designs.

7. *Arithmetic*—A series of calculation problems which the patient solves with paper and pencil, ranging from simple arithmetic to algebra and calculus depending on ability.

8. *Object Assembly*—The patient assembles puzzles of familiar objects. (Not part of the WPPSI.)

9. *Comprehension*—The patient is asked to describe the meaning of proverbs, method of solving problems, and other simple tests of reasoning and judgment.

10. *Digit Symbol*—This is a coding task in which the patient is asked to write the appropriate symbol from a key beneath the paired number or letter. (Not part of the WPPSI.)

11. *Similarities*—The patient is asked to form associations between multiple pairs of objects, for example, "How are a table and a bookcase alike?"

Additional WISC-R and WPPSI subtests:

12. *Mazes*—This subtest is optional for use on the WISC-R and WPPSI. The patient is asked to solve a series of progressively more difficult mazes.

13. *Animal House*—This subtest is used on the WPPSI in place of the Digit Symbol coding task. The child must match a colored cylinder with an animal's picture.

14. *Geometric Design*—A WPPSI subtest in which the child copies simple figures.

15. *Sentences*—This subtest is for optional use on the WPPSI. It is a memory task which replaces the Digit Span.

References used for Psychological Testing section:

Anastasi A: Psychological Testing, 6th Edition. New York, Macmillan, 1988

Mitchell JV Jr (ed): The Ninth Mental Measurements Yearbook, Vols 1 and 2. Buros Institute of Mental Measurements. Lincoln, NE, University of Nebraska Press, 1985

Sweetland RC, Keyser DJ (eds): Tests: A Comprehensive Reference for Assessments in Psychology, Education, and Business, 2nd Edition. Kansas City, MO, Test Corporation of America, 1986

MEDICAL PSYCHIATRY

SOME CLUES SUGGESTIVE OF ORGANIC MENTAL DISORDER

    I.   Psychiatric symptom onset after the age of 40 years
   II.   Psychiatric symptoms begin. . .
       A. During a major illness
       B. While taking drugs known to cause mental symptoms
       C. Suddenly, in a patient without prior psychiatric history or known stressors
  III.   History of . . .
       A. Alcohol or drug abuse
       B. Physical illness impairing major organ function
       C. Taking multiple prescribed or over-the-counter drugs
       D. History of poor response to apparently adequate psychiatric treatment
  IV.   Family history of. . .
       A. Degenerative or inheritable brain disease
       B. Metabolic disease (e.g., diabetes, pernicious anemia)

V. Mental signs include. . .
  A. Altered level of consciousness
  B. Fluctuating mental status
  C. Cognitive impairment
  D. Episodic, recurrent, or cyclic course
  E. Visual, tactile, or olfactory hallucinations
VI. Physical signs include. . .
  A. Signs of organ malfunction that can affect the brain
  B. Focal neurologic deficits
  C. Diffuse subcortical dysfunction (e.g., slowed speech, mentation or movement; ataxia, incoordination; tremor, chorea, asterixis, dysarthria)
  D. Cortical dysfunction (e.g., dysphasia, apraxias, agnosias, visuospatial deficits, or defective cortical sensation)

Modified from Hoffman RS, Koran LM: Detecting physical illness in patients with mental disorders. Psychosomatics 25:654–660, 1984.

DIFFERENTIAL DIAGNOSIS OF THE DEMENTIA SYNDROME

Primary Degenerative Dementia:
   Alzheimer's disease
   Pick's Disease
Multi-infarct Dementia
Intracranial Space-Occupying Lesions:
   Intracranial neoplasms
   Normal pressure hydrocephalus
   Subdural hematoma
Depression With "Pseudodementia"

DIFFERENTIAL DIAGNOSIS OF THE DEMENTIA SYNDROME—continued

Toxic and Metabolic Disturbances:
  Chemical exposures (heavy metals, organic solvents)
  Drug intoxications (alcoholic dementia most common type)
  Endocrinopathies
  Infections (e.g., AIDS, neurosyphilis, tuberculosis, other bacterial, viral, or fungal meningitides)
  Inflammatory disturbances
  Nutritional deficiencies (e.g., B_{12}, folate)
  Systemic illnesses (e.g., giant cell arteritis, systemic lupus erythematosus)
Extrapyramidal Syndromes Associated With Dementia:
  Huntington's disease
  Parkinson's disease
  Progressive supranuclear palsy
  Spinocerebellar dementia
  Wilson's disease
Posttraumatic Dementia

Modified from Cummings JL: Dementia: definition, classification, and differential diagnosis. Psychiatr Ann 14:85–89, 1984.

LABORATORY SCREEN FOR ORGANIC BRAIN SYNDROME

Suggested for All Psychiatric Hospital Admissions:
Hematology group (hemoglobin, hematocrit, leukocyte count, platelets)
Chemistry group (electrolytes, liver function tests, glucose, calcium, renal function tests)
Serum B_{12} / folate
Syphilis serology
Thyroid function tests (total T4, TSH, T3 uptake)
Erythrocyte sedimentation rate
Urinalysis

If Alcoholism Is Suspected, Add:
γ-Glutamyltransferase (GGT)
Triglycerides
Erythrocyte indices (mean corpuscular volume)

Consider, Depending on Presentation:
Blood:
    Human immunodeficiency virus (HIV) antibody screen
    Blood alcohol level
    Drug levels of psychopharmacologic agents
    Serum copper and ceruloplasmin

Urine:
    Urine drug abuse survey
    24-hour urine levels of lead, mercury, and arsenic
    24-hour urine levels for quantitative porphyrins
    Urinary metanephrines/5-hydroxyindoleacetic acid (5-HIAA)

Imaging:
    Computed tomography (CT) of head
    Magnetic resonance imaging (MRI) of head
    Chest radiograph

Other:
    Electroencephalogram (EEG)
    Evoked potentials
    Electrocardiogram (EKG)
    Cerebral spinal fluid (CSF) examination
    Neuropsychological testing

For Nutritionally Depleted Patients, Consider:
    Zinc, copper, carotene, iron, or serum transferrin levels
    Basal metabolic rate
    Triiodothyronine (T3), thyroid-stimulating hormone (TSH)
    Total serum protein, albumin/globulin ratio

MEDICAL CONDITIONS MANIFESTING AS PSYCHIATRIC DISORDERS

The following is a list of medical disorders that are commonly associated with psychiatric symptoms. The list has been selected to emphasize those disorders that are most often considered in a psychiatric differential diagnosis. Drugs that cause psychiatric symptoms are listed in separate tables later in this section of the book.

Sources:

Hurst JW (ed): Medicine for the Practicing Physician, 2nd Edition. Boston, MA, Butterworths, 1988

Braunwald E, Isselbacher KJ, Petersdorf RG, et al (eds): Harrison's Principles of Internal Medicine, 11th Edition. New York, McGraw-Hill, 1987

*Common = 100–1,000/100,000; infrequent = 10–100/100,000; rare = <10/100,000.

Disorder (alternate name) Prevalence range* Age at onset Sex ratio	Signs or symptoms	Psychiatric features	Comments
Medical Category			
Connective Tissue Diseases			
Giant cell arteritis (temporal arteritis) Incidence: infrequent in persons age 50+ yr 50+ yr Females 2:1	Headache, joint/muscle pain, low-grade fever, vision loss	Depression, confusion	Rapid diagnosis and treatment may prevent blindness

	Physical Signs	Psychiatric Symptoms	Comments
Systemic lupus erythematosus Infrequent 20–40 yr Females 10:1	Arthritis, malar rash, lymphadenopathy, oral ulcers, fever, weight loss	Depression, memory impairment, delirium, psychosis	Treatment with corticosteroids may complicate psychiatric features

Endocrine/Metabolic

	Physical Signs	Psychiatric Symptoms	Comments
Hyperadrenalism (Cushing's syndrome) Common; multiple causes 30–50 yr Females 3:1	Central obesity, moon facies, striae, weakness, acne	Depression, lability, anxiety, somatic delusions, psychosis	Clinical picture varies with etiology
Adrenal cortical insufficiency (Addison's disease) Rare Any age Both sexes	Hyperpigmentation, orthostatic hypotension, anorexia, dizziness	Depression, apathy, paranoia, psychosis	Insidious onset may resemble depression, psychasthenia; many etiologies
Hyperparathyroidism Common 50–60 yr Females > males	Hypercalcemia, weight loss, constipation, dyspepsia, renal stones	Depression, anxiety, confusion, irritability, toxic psychosis	Most individuals asymptomatic with high Ca^{2+} detected by laboratory examination
Hypoparathyroidism ... Any age Both sexes	Hypercalcemia, dry skin, diarrhea, congestive heart failure, extrapyramidal symptoms, tetany	Irritability, paranoia, depression, delirium, psychosis	Iatrogenic form (postsurgery) is most common

MEDICAL CONDITIONS MANIFESTING AS PSYCHIATRIC DISORDERS—continued

Disorder (alternate name) Prevalence range* Age at onset Sex ratio	Signs or symptoms	Psychiatric features	Comments
Hyperthyroidism Common Graves'; 30–40 yr; toxic multinodular goiter: 50 + yr Females 10:1	Tremor, weight loss, palpitations, warm/moist skin	Anxiety, depression, irritability, grandiosity, psychosis	Rapid onset resembles anxiety; slow onset associated with depression
Hypothyroidism (myxedema) Infrequent Adolescents, adults Females 5:1	Dry skin, cold intolerance, constipation, slow/hoarse speech	Impaired cognition, somnolence, anxiety, irritability, somatic delusions, paranoia, hallucinations	Slow onset may be mistaken for depression or sleep apnea
Hypoglycemia Multiple causes Any age Both sexes	Headache, diaphoresis, tremor	Anxiety, irritability, confusion, obtundation	Symptoms occur in fasting or postprandial states in which hypoglycemia may occur

Syndrome of inappropriate secretion of antidiuretic hormone (SIADH) (water intoxication) Multiple causes Any age Both sexes	Hyponatremia, headache, anorexia, weakness	Irritability, obtundation, delirium	Multiple etiologies

Gastrointestinal

Hepatolenticular degeneration (Wilson's disease) Infrequent Mean age: 15 yr Both sexes	Abdominal pain, tremor, ataxia, Kayser-Fleischer ring	Irritability, depression, delusions, dementia	Autosomal recessive; psychiatric symptoms may precede other findings

Hematologic

Acute intermittent porphyria Rare Adolescents, young adults Females > males	Abdominal pain, vomiting, peripheral neuropathy, sensory loss	Mood change, psychosis, delirium	Autosomal dominant; SIADH may occur; attack provoked by anesthetics, sedatives, hypnotics, other drugs

MEDICAL CONDITIONS MANIFESTING AS PSYCHIATRIC DISORDERS—continued

Disorder (alternate name) Prevalence range* Age at onset Sex ratio	Signs or symptoms	Psychiatric features	Comments
		Infectious	
AIDS-related dementia May be common among AIDS patients High-risk groups of any age Males > females	Fever, weight loss, lymphadenopathy	Depression, irritability, paranoia, psychosis, dementia	Dementia may be complicated by infectious agents, toxic/metabolic conditions, or neoplasms
Tuberculous meningitis 5% of U.S. TB patients Children, elderly Both sexes	Low-grade fever, weight loss, headache, meningeal signs	Obtundation, dementia	Insidious onset; CNS signs may be mild; TB more common among poor, alcoholic
Neurosyphilis (general paresis) Rare Adults Males 4:1	None or headache, papilledema, slapping gait, Argyll Robertson pupil	Personality change, confusion, irritability, depression, delusions, dementia	Insidious onset
Cryptococcal meningitis Rare Adults Males > females	Headache, nausea, dizziness, clumsiness	Impaired cognition, personality change, obtundation	2/3 patients are immuno-compromised; pigeons are biologic vector; insidious onset

Creutzfeldt-Jakob disease Rare 52 yr Both sexes	Myoclonic jerks, visual disturbances	Rapidly progressive dementia	EEG is diagnostic

Neoplasias

Pancreatic carcinoma Infrequent 50–70 yr Males 3:1	Abdominal pain that radiates to back, weight loss, jaundice	Depression, apathy	Insidious onset with few physical findings initially
Pheochromocytoma Rare Any age Both sexes	Hypertension, headache, sweating, palpitations	Anxiety	0.1% of hypertensive patients

Neurologic

Intracranial tumors Rare Any age Both sexes	None or papilledema, headache, vomiting, focal neurologic signs	Depression, anxiety, personality change, obtundation	Clinical picture varies with lesion
Subdural hematoma Common, especially in alcoholics Adults Males > females	Headache	Irritability, confusion, depression, dementia	50% of patients lack history of head trauma; a treatable cause of dementia

MEDICAL CONDITIONS MANIFESTING AS PSYCHIATRIC DISORDERS—continued

Disorder (alternate name) Prevalence range* Age at onset Sex ratio	Signs or symptoms	Psychiatric features	Comments
Communicating hydrocephalus (normal pressure hydrocephalus)			
7% of dementia patients 45+ yr Both sexes	Gait ataxia, urinary incontinence	Apathy, psychomotor retardation, dementia	A treatable cause of dementia
Seizure disorders (epilepsy)			
Common Any age Both sexes	Varies; staring, automatisms, sensory aura, jerking	Postictal confusion, personality changes interictally	Must differentiate from hysteria; conversion symptom, daydreaming, rage attacks
Postconcussion syndrome			
Unknown Any age Both sexes	Headache, dizziness, insomnia, seizure	Irritability, personality change, depression	Symptoms may follow minor head trauma and persist for years
Alzheimer's type dementia (senile dementia)			
5% of persons age 65 65–70 yr Both sexes	None until late stage	Irritability, personality change, depression, dementia	Insidious onset; incidence increases with age
Multi-infarct dementia			
10%–15% of dementia patients ... Male > female	Focal neurologic signs, hypertension	Lability, personality change, dementia	Stepwise progression of impairment

Peripheral neuropathy Common Middle-aged and elderly more common Both sexes	Numbness, pain, ataxias, atrophy of skin or muscle of extremities	Vague complaints	May be confused with hypochondriasis or somatization disorder
Multiple sclerosis Infrequent 10–55 yr Female 3:2	Focal neurologic deficits, paresthesias, clumsiness, optic neuritis	Affective disturbance, memory loss, paroxysmal sensory or motor disorder	Episodic course with long latent periods; may be mistaken for somatization
Myasthenia gravis Rare <40 yr Female 3:1; elderly 1:1	Diplopia, ptosis, dysphagia, weakness after exertion	Anxiety from respiratory muscle weakness & hypoxia, depression	Diurnal pattern (best in A.M.) is distinct from depression; sedatives, tranquilizers, and anticonvulsants may exacerbate
Parkinson's disease Common 55 yr Males 3:2	Resting tremor, rigidity, bradykinesia, loss of postural reflexes	Depression, dependency, dementia, psychosis	Insidious onset; drugs may induce psychosis; depression may complicate picture

MEDICAL CONDITIONS MANIFESTING AS PSYCHIATRIC DISORDERS—continued

Disorder (alternate name) Prevalence range* Age at onset Sex ratio	Signs or symptoms	Psychiatric features	Comments
Huntington's disease Rare 35–45 yr Both sexes	Chorea	Personality change, irritability, cognitive decline, depression, dementia	Autosomal dominant inheritance; suicide is frequent
Nutritional			
Pernicious anemia (vitamin B₁₂ deficiency) Rare 60+ yr Both sexes	Ataxia, peripheral neuropathy, macrocytic anemia, sore tongue	Depression, paranoia, irritability, dementia	Insidious onset; mental status changes may precede anemia; more common among northern Europeans
Folate deficiency Rare Poor, alcoholics, women of childbearing age	Anemia	Insomnia, irritability, depression, memory disturbance	Psychiatric symptoms may precede anemia

*Common = 100–1,000/100,000; infrequent = 10–100/100,000; rare = <10/100,000.

SPECIFIC TESTS FOR ORGANIC MENTAL DISORDERS

Probable cause	Tests
Endocrine Abnormalities:	
Thyroid disease	Serum triiodothyronine (T3), total thyroxine (T4), thyroid-stimulating hormone (TSH), thyrotropin-releasing hormone (TRH) stimulation test, thyroid imaging studies
Parathyroid	Serum calcium and phosphorus, parathyroid hormone (PTH)
Adrenal	Serum cortisol, urine cortisol, imaging studies, challenge tests
Pancreas	Serum glucose, glucose tolerance test, amylase, hemoglobin A_{1c}
Metabolic Disturbances:	
Liver disease	Serum ammonia, aspartate aminotransferase (AST/SGOT), alanine aminotransferase (ALT/SGPT), bilirubin, imaging studies, liver biopsy
Porphyria	Urine porphyrins
Pulmonary disease	PO_2, PCO_2, acid-base balance, chest radiograph, pulmonary function studies
Renal disease	Serum electrolytes, creatinine, urea nitrogen (BUN), magnesium, calcium, acid-base balance, osmolality, urinalysis, serum protein and albumin, imaging studies, biopsy

SPECIFIC TESTS FOR ORGANIC MENTAL DISORDERS—continued

Probable cause	Tests
Syndrome of inappropriate secretion of antidiuretic hormone (SIADH)	Serum osmolality, urine osmolality, serum sodium
Hepatolenticular degeneration (Wilson's disease)	Serum copper, ceruloplasmin, urinary copper, slit-lamp examination

Nutritional and Deficiency States:

Probable cause	Tests
Pernicious anemia	Serum vitamin B_{12}, erythrocyte indices, peripheral blood smear
Folic acid deficiency	Serum folate, erythrocyte indices, peripheral blood smear
Wernicke-Korsakoff's syndrome	Liver function tests, erythrocyte indices, triglycerides

Neurologic:

Probable cause	Tests
Multiple sclerosis	CSF examination for gamma globulins and oligoclonal bands, high-resolution computed tomographic (CT) scan or magnetic resonance imaging (MRI), visual-evoked responses
Myasthenia gravis	Acetylcholine receptor binding antibody
Epilepsy	Electroencephalogram (sleep-deprived)
Normal pressure hydrocephaly	CT scan
Dementia (unknown cause)	Chemistry group, complete blood cell count, erythrocyte sedimentation rate, urinalysis, thyroid function tests, B_{12}, CSF examination, CT or MRI scan, electroencephalogram

Infectious:

Brain abscess, encephalitis, meningitis, subacute bacterial endocarditis

Blood cultures, leukocyte count and differential; serologic tests for fungi, syphilis; viral antibody titers (HIV); CSF examination for protein, glucose, cell count, cytology, serologies, pathogen culture; electroencephalogram, brain imaging

Connective Tissue Disease:

Systemic lupus erythematosus

Erythrocyte sedimentation rate, lupus erythematosus clot, antinuclear antibody, peripheral blood smear (rouleau formation), cerebrospinal fluid examination

Giant cell arteritis

Erythrocyte sedimentation rate, temporal artery biopsy

Traumatic:

Postconcussion syndrome

Brain imaging studies, skull films, electroencephalogram

Fat embolism

Urinalysis (lipuria), funduscopic examination, brain imaging

Drug or Medication Toxicity:

Lead, mercury, thallium, arsenic

Peripheral smear, blood cell count, erythrocyte indices, 24-h urine for heavy metals

Carbon monoxide

Carboxyhemoglobin

Organophosphate insecticides

Serum cholinesterase

DRUGS THAT CAUSE PSYCHIATRIC SYMPTOMS

DRUGS THAT MAY INDUCE ANXIETY

Anticholinergics and Antihistamines
Antidepressants
  Fluoxetine
  Monoamine oxidase inhibitors
  Tricyclic antidepressants (especially early in therapy)
Benzodiazepines (Paradoxical reaction; withdrawal states)
Euphoriants and Hallucinogens
  Cannabis
  Lysergide (LSD), mescaline, psilocybin
  Phencyclidine (PCP)
Hormones
  Androgens, estrogens, progesterones
  Corticosteroids
  Thyroid supplements
Neuroleptics (akathisia)
Stimulants and Sympathomimetics
  Amphetamines
  Methylphenidate, pemoline
  Ephedrine, pseudoephedrine, phenylpropanolamine
  Xanthines: caffeine, theobromine, theophylline
Withdrawal States
  Especially from alcohol, sedatives, narcotics
Others
  Cycloserine
  Metrizamide
  Quinacrine

DRUGS THAT MAY INDUCE DEPRESSION

Antiarrhythmics
  Digitalis
  Disopyramide
  Nifedipine
Anticonvulsants
Antihypertensives
  Clonidine
  Guanethidine
  Hydralazine
  Methyldopa

  Prazosin
  Propranolol (? other β-blockers)
  Reserpine
  Trichlormethiazide

Antimicrobials
  Cycloserine
  Isoniazid
  Metronidazole
  Nalidixic acid
Chemotherapeutic Agents
  Asparaginase
  Vinblastine, vincristine
Hormone Preparations
  Corticosteroids
  Oral contraceptives
  Thyroid supplements
Nonsteroidal Anti-inflammatory Drugs
Sedative Agents
  Alcohol
  Barbiturates

  Benzodiazepines
  Hypnotics

Withdrawal States
  Especially from cocaine and other stimulants
Other
  Cimetidine, ranitidine
  Disulfiram
  Levodopa, carbidopa
  Metoclopramide
  Metrizamide

DRUGS THAT MAY INDUCE DELIRIUM, HALLUCINATIONS, OR PARANOIA

Antiarrhythmics
  Digitalis, lidocaine, procainamide, quinacrine
Anticholinergics
Anticonvulsants
Antidepressants (tricyclics)
Antimicrobials, antiparasitics, antivirals
  Amantadine
  Amphotericin B, metronidazole
  Thiabendazole
  Cycloserine, isoniazid
  Chloroquine, hydroxychloroquine
  Dapsone
  Procaine penicillin
Antihistamines
  Including H_2 blockers: cimetidine, ranitidine
β-Adrenergic Blockers
Chemotherapeutic Agents (especially intrathecal administration)
  Asparaginase, cisplatin, vincristine
Euphoriants and Hallucinogens
  Cannabis, lysergide (LSD), mescaline, psilocybin, phencyclidine
  (PCP)
Hormone Preparations
  Corticosteroids
Nonsteroidal Anti-inflammatory Agents
Sedatives
  Alcohol, benzodiazepines, barbiturates, hypnotics
Stimulants and Sympathomimetics
  Amphetamines, cocaine, methylphenidate, pemoline, sympatho-
  mimetics
Withdrawal States
  Especially from alcohol and sedatives: delirium tremens
Other

Albuterol	Levodopa, carbidopa
Bromides	Methyldopa
Bromocriptine	Methysergide
Disulfiram	Metrizamide

SEXUAL DYSFUNCTION ASSOCIATED WITH DRUG THERAPY

The Medical Letter on Drugs and Therapeutics includes references to case reports.

Drug	Adverse effect
Acetazolamide (Diamox)	Loss of libido; decreased potency
Alprazolam (Xanax)	Inhibition of orgasm; delayed or no ejaculation
Amiloride (Midamor)	Impotence; decreased libido
Amiodarone (Cordarone)	Decreased libido
Amitriptyline (Elavil)	Loss of libido; impotence; no ejaculation
Amoxapine (Asendin)	Loss of libido; impotence; retrograde, painful, or no ejaculation
Amphetamines and related anorexic drugs*	Chronic abuse: impotence; delayed or no ejaculation in men; no orgasm in women
Anticholinergics†	Impotence
Atenolol (Tenormin)	Impotence
Baclofen (Lioresal)	Impotence; inability to ejaculate
Barbiturates	Decreased libido; impotence
Carbamazepine (Tegretol)	Impotence
Chlorpromazine (Thorazine)	Decreased libido; impotence; no ejaculation; priapism
Chlorprothixene (Taractan)	Inhibition of ejaculation; decreased intensity of orgasm
Chlorthalidone (Hygroton)	Decreased libido; impotence
Cimetidine (Tagamet)	Decreased libido (men and women); impotence
Clofibrate (Atromid-S)	Decreased libido; impotence
Clomipramine (Anafranil)	Decreased libido (men and women); impotence; retarded or no ejaculation (men) or orgasm (women); spontaneous orgasm associated with yawning
Clonidine (Catapres)	Impotence; delayed or retrograde ejaculation; inhibition of orgasm (women)
Danazol (Danocrine)	Increased or decreased libido
Desipramine (Norpramin)	Decreased libido; impotence; difficult ejaculation and painful orgasm

SEXUAL DYSFUNCTION ASSOCIATED WITH DRUG THERAPY—continued

Drug	Adverse effect
Diazepam (Valium)	Decreased libido; delayed ejaculation; retarded or no orgasm in women
Dichlorphenamide (Daranide)	Decreased libido; impotence
Digoxin	Decreased libido; impotence
Disopyramide (Norpace)	Impotence
Disulfiram (Antabuse)	Impotence
Doxepin (Adapin; Sinequan)	Decreased libido; ejaculatory dysfunction
Estrogens	Decreased libido in men
Ethionamide (Trecator-SC)	Impotence
Ethosuximide (Zarontin)	Increased libido
Ethoxzolamide (Ethamide)	Decreased libido
Fenfluramine (Pondimin)	Loss of libido (frequent in women with large doses or long-term use); impotence
Fluphenazine (Prolixin; Permitil)	Changes in libido; erection difficulties; inhibition of ejaculation
Guanabenz (Wytensin)	Impotence
Guanadrel (Hylorel)	Decreased libido; delayed or retrograde ejaculation; impotence
Guanethidine (Ismelin)	Decreased libido; impotence; delayed, retrograde, or no ejaculation
Haloperidol (Haldol)	Impotence; painful ejaculation
Hydralazine (Apresoline)	Impotence; priapism
Hydroxyprogesterone caproate (Delalutin)	Impotence
Imipramine (Tofranil)	Decreased libido; impotence; painful, delayed ejaculation; delayed orgasm in women
Indapamide (Lozol)	Decreased libido; impotence
Interferon (Roferon-A)	Decreased libido; impotence
Isocarboxazid (Marplan)	Impotence; delayed ejaculation; no orgasm (women)
Ketoconazole (Nizoral)	Impotence

Drug	Adverse effect
Labetalol (Trandate; Normodyne)	Priapism; impotence; delayed or no ejaculation; decreased libido
Levodopa (Dopar)	Increased libido
Lithium (Eskalith)	Decreased libido; impotence
Maprotiline (Ludiomil)	Impotence; decreased libido
Mazindol (Sanorex; Mazanor)	Impotence; spontaneous ejaculation; painful testes
Mecamylamine (Inversine)	Impotence; decreased libido
Mepenzolate bromide (Cantil)	Impotence
Mesoridazine (Serentil)	No ejaculation; impotence; priapism
Methadone (Dolophine)	Decreased libido; impotence; no orgasm (men and women); retarded ejaculation
Methandrostenolone (Dianabol)	Decreased libido
Methantheline bromide (Banthine)	Impotence
Methazolamide (Neptazane)	Decreased libido (men and women); impotence
Methyldopa (Aldomet)	Decreased libido (men and women); impotence; delayed or no ejaculation (men) or orgasm (women)
Metoclopramide (Reglan)	Impotence; decreased libido
Metoprolol (Lopressor)	Decreased libido; impotence
Metyrosine (Demser)	Impotence; failure of ejaculation
Mexiletine (Mexitil)	Impotence; decreased libido
Molindone (Moban)	Priapism
Naltrexone (Trexan)	Delayed ejaculation; decreased potency
Naproxen (Anaprox; Naprosyn)	Impotence; no ejaculation
Norethandrolone	Decreased libido; impotence
Norethindrone (Norlutin)	Decreased libido; impotence

SEXUAL DYSFUNCTION ASSOCIATED WITH DRUG THERAPY—continued

Drug	Adverse effect
Nortriptyline (Aventyl; Pamelor)	Impotence; decreased libido
Pargyline (Eutonyl)	No ejaculation; impotence
Perphenazine (Trilafon)	Decreased or no ejaculation
Phenelzine (Nardil)	Impotence; retarded or no ejaculation; delayed or no orgasm (men and women)
Phenytoin (Dilantin)	Decreased libido; impotence
Pimozide (Orap)	Impotence; no ejaculation; decreased libido
Pindolol (Visken)	Impotence
Prazosin (Minipress)	Impotence; priapism
Primidone (Mysoline)	Decreased libido; impotence
Progesterone	Decreased libido; impotence
Propantheline bromide (Pro-Banthine)	Impotence
Propranolol (Inderal)	Loss of libido (men and women); impotence
Protriptyline (Vivactil)	Loss of libido; impotence; painful ejaculation
Ranitidine (Zantac)	Loss of libido; impotence
Reserpine	Decreased libido (men and women); impotence; decreased or no ejaculation
Spironolactone (Aldactone)	Decreased libido (men and women); impotence
Thiazide diuretics	Impotence
Thioridazine (Mellaril)	Impotence; priapism; delayed, decreased, painful, retrograde, or no ejaculation
Thiothixene (Navane)	Spontaneous ejaculation; impotence; priapism
Timolol (Blocadren; Timolide; Timoptic)	Decreased libido (men and women); impotence
Tranylcypromine (Parnate)	Impotence
Trazodone (Desyrel)	Priapism; increased libido (women); retrograde ejaculation

Drug	Adverse effect
Trifluoperazine (Stelazine)	Decreased, painful, or no ejaculation; spontaneous ejaculation
Verapamil (Calan)	Impotence

*Diethylpropion (Tenuate; Tepanil); phendimetrazine (Plegine); phenmetrazine (Preludin); phentermine (Fastin).
†Anisotropine (Valpin); dicyclomine (Bentyl); glycopyrrolate (Robinul); homatropine methylbromide (Mesopin); oxybutinin (Ditropan); tridihexethyl chloride (Pathilon); clidinium (Quarzan); hexocyclium (Tral).
From Drugs that cause sexual dysfunction. Med Lett Drugs Ther 29:65–70, 1987. By permission of The Medical Letter.

SCREENING FOR DRUGS IN SERUM AND URINE

The following is a list of drug assays that are available at most large medical laboratories. In general, screening for drugs in urine is more sensitive than serum screening but results are qualitative. For quantitative results, specific serum testing must be done. Physicians are advised to check with their laboratory director for the availability of specific tests and the type and amount of specimen required. In ordering any test of this type, physicians should supply information to the laboratory as to drugs patients are known or suspected to have ingested, with the amount and time of ingestion, if known. This information may permit customizing the assay for more accurate testing.

Drug screening differs from therapeutic drug monitoring. If a specific drug level or assay is required, that test should be ordered rather than a drug screen.

THE DRUG SCREEN

The drug screen assay is a specific test for a limited number of compounds. Drugs are detected in body fluids (urine, serum, gastric) in the drug screen assay. Generally, drugs detected in the serum drug screen assay will be detected in gastric fluid and urine as well, but results can be quantified only for serum. Drugs not included in the table are not detected in the drug screen assay. Detectability is a function of the laboratory method, dose and time of ingestion, and half-life of the drug.

	Urine	Serum	Detected — Serum, only at toxic concentrations	Not detectable (ND) or special assay (SA) required
Analgesics				
Acetaminophen (Tylenol)	+	+		
Acetylsalicylic acid (aspirin)	+	+		
Ibuprofen (Motrin, Advil, Nuprin)	+	+		
Meperidine (Demerol)	+			
Methadone (Dolophine)	+			
Naproxen (Naprosyn)	+	+		
Opiates	+			
Pentazocine (Talwin)	+			
Phenacetin	+	+		
Phenylbutazone (Butazolidin)	+	+		
Propoxyphene (Darvon)	+	+		
Salicylic acid	+			
Anticonvulsants (other than barbiturates)				
Carbamazepine (Tegretol)	+	+		
Ethosuximide (Zarontin)	+	+		
Methsuximide (Celontin)	+	+		
Phenytoin (Dilantin)	+	+		
Valproic acid (Depakene)	+	+		

| | Detected | | | Not detectable (ND) or special assay (SA) required |
	Urine	Serum	Serum, only at toxic concentrations	
Antidepressants				
Amitriptyline (Elavil)	+		+	
Amoxapine (Asendin)	+		+	
Desipramine (Norpramin)	+		+	
Doxepin (Sinequan)	+		+	
Imipramine (Tofranil)	+		+	
Fluoxetine (Prozac)				SA
Maprotiline (Ludiomil)	+		+	
Nortriptyline (Aventyl)	+		+	
Protriptyline (Vivactil)	+		+	
Trazodone (Desyrel)				ND
Trimipramine (Surmontil)	+		+	
Antihistamines				
Brompheniramine	+			
Chlorpheniramine (Chlor-Trimeton)	+			
Diphenhydramine (Benadryl)	+			
Doxylamine (Unisom)	+			
Thonzylamine	+			
Antipsychotics				
Chlorpromazine (Thorazine)	+		+	
Haloperidol (Haldol)				SA
Prochlorperazine (Compazine)	+			
Thioridazine (Mellaril)	+		+	
Trifluoperazine (Stelazine)	+			
Serum phenothiazine screen				SA

THE DRUG SCREEN—continued

| | Detected | | | Not detectable (ND) or special assay (SA) required |
	Urine	Serum	Serum, only at toxic concentrations	
Barbiturates				
Allobarbital	+	+		
Amobarbital (Amytal)	+	+		
Aprobarbital (Alurate)	+	+		
Barbital	+	+		
Butabarbital (Butisol)	+	+		
Butalbital (Fiorinal)	+	+		
Mephobarbital (Mebaral)	+	+		
Metharbital (Gemonil)	+	+		
Pentobarbital (Nembutal)	+	+		
Primidone (Mysoline)	+	+		
Phenobarbital	+	+		
Secobarbital (Seconal)	+	+		
Thiopental (Pentothal)	+	+		
Benzodiazepines				
Chlordiazepoxide (Librium)	SA	+		
Diazepam (Valium)	SA	+		
Flurazepam (Dalmane)	SA	+		
Nordiazepam (metabolite of Tranxene)	SA	+		
Oxazepam (Serax)	SA	+		
Diuretics				SA

| | Detected | | Not detectable (ND) or special assay (SA) required |
	Urine	Serum	Serum, only at toxic concentrations	

	Urine	Serum	Serum, only at toxic concentrations	ND or SA required
Hypoglycemics (sulfonylureas)				
Acetohexamine (Dymelor)	+	+		
Chlorpropamide (Diabinese)	+	+		
Tolazamide (Tolinase)	+	+		
Tolbutamide (Orinase)	+	+		
Lithium				SA
Monoamine Oxidase Inhibitors (MAOIs)				SA
Sedatives (other than barbiturates or benzodiazepines)				
Carisoprodol (Soma)	+	+		
Chloral hydrate				SA
Ethchlorvynol (Placidyl)	+	+		
Glutethimide (Doriden)	+	+		
Meprobamate (Miltown)	+	+		
Methaqualone (Quaalude)	+	+		
Methyprylon (Noludar)	+	+		
Stimulants				
Amphetamine (Benzedrine)	+			
Caffeine	+	+		
Cocaine	+			
Methamphetamine (Desoxyn)	+			
Methylphenidate (Ritalin)	+			
Nicotine	+		+	
Phencyclidine	+			
Phenylpropanolamine (Dexatrim)	+			
Strychnine	+		+	

THE DRUG SCREEN—continued

	Detected			Not detectable (ND) or special assay (SA) required
	Urine	Serum	Serum, only at toxic concentrations	
Theobromine (cacao bean products, tea)	+	+		
Theophylline (aminophylline)	+	+		
Sympathomimetics				
dl-Ephedrine	+			
THC (tetrahydrocannabinol)/ marijuana	+			
Others				
Dextromethorphan	+			
Disopyramide (Norpace)	+	+		
Lidocaine (Xylocaine)	+	+		
Lysergic acid diethylamide (LSD)				ND
Penicillin metabolites	+			
Trimethoprim	+			

SCREENING FOR DRUGS OF ABUSE

Drug Abuse Survey: Useful as a quick screen for the presence of major categories of drugs of abuse. Urine test for alcohol, amphetamines, barbiturates, benzodiazepines, cocaine, opiates, phencyclidine, and tetrahydrocannabinol by class with an immunoassay or thin-layer chromatography procedure. Results are presumptive since no confirmation is performed.

Drug Abuse Survey With Confirmation: A urine test for the same drugs as the Drug Abuse Survey, but this assay combines gas chromatography–mass spectrometry (GC-MS) to confirm the results of the screening assay. This is a much more accurate and sensitive test, and it is quantitative but more expensive than the Drug Abuse Survey. GC-MS may be used to test body fluids other than urine. This assay is recommended for employee screening programs or situations in which accuracy is paramount. Specimens should be collected under observation for greater reliability. Some states require that specimens collected for employee screening or forensic purposes be accompanied by documentation showing the chain of custody for each specimen.

Detectability of drugs in urine or serum varies with the amount, time and route of consumption, chronicity of use, and the technique and skill of the testing laboratory. For GC-MS, limits of detectability are as follows.

Drug	Amount/ml	Approximate duration of detectability (days)*
Alcohol	300 μg	1
Amphetamines	500 ng	2
Barbiturates	1,000 ng	1–3
Benzodiazepines	300 ng	3
Cocaine	150 ng	2–3
Opiates	300 ng	2
Phencyclidine	25 ng	8
Tetrahydrocannabinol carboxylic acid	<15 ng	3–20

*May vary widely depending on amount ingested, compound, physical state of subject, and other factors. Modified from Council on Scientific Affairs, The American Medical Association: Scientific issues in drug testing. JAMA 257:3110–3114, 1987.
See also: Gold MS, Dackis CA: Role of the laboratory in the evaluation of suspected drug abuse. J Clin Psychiatry 47 (suppl): 17–23, 1986.

DRUGS THAT MAY INTERFERE WITH THE DRUG ABUSE SURVEY

Test substance	Possible cross-reactors
Amphetamines	Diethylpropion
	Dopamine
	Ephedrine
	Fenfluramine
	p-Hydroxyamphetamine
	Isoxsuprine
	l-Methamphetamine
	Methylphenidate
	Nylidrin
	Phentermine
	Phenylephrine
	Phenylpropanolamine
	Propylhexedrine
	Pseudoephedrine
Barbiturates	Glutethimide
	Phenytoin
Opiates	Chlorpromazine
	Codeine
	Dextromethorphan
	Diphenoxylate
	Hydromorphone
	Meperidine
	Oxycodone
	d-Propoxyphene
Phencyclidine	Chlorpromazine
	Dextromethorphan
	Diphenhydramine
	Doxylamine
	Meperidine
	Thioridazine

From Council on Scientific Affairs: Scientific issues in drug testing. JAMA 257:3110–3114, 1987. By permission of the American Medical Association.

INDICATIONS FOR CEREBRAL IMAGING OF PSYCHIATRIC PATIENTS

1. Confusion or dementia of unknown cause
2. First episode of psychotic disorder of unknown origin
3. Movement disorder of unknown origin
4. Anorexia nervosa, especially if atypical presentation
5. Prolonged catatonia
6. First episode of major affective disorder or personality change after age 50 years
7. Prior to lumbar puncture if increased intracranial pressure is suspected
8. Presence of unexplained neurologic findings

Modified from Weinberger DR: Brain disease and psychiatric illness: when should a psychiatrist order a CAT scan? Am J Psychiatry 141:1521–1527, 1984.
See also: Andreasen NC: Brain imaging: applications in psychiatry. Science 239:1381–1388, 1988.

COMPARISON OF COMPUTED TOMOGRAPHY (CT) AND MAGNETIC RESONANCE IMAGING (MRI)

CT is generally adequate to screen for organic causes of psychiatric symptoms and is better tolerated by confused or agitated patients because of the shorter scanning time. MRI may be preferable when higher resolution is required or to image certain brain regions.

	CT	MRI
Ionizing radiation	Yes	No
Resolution	0.5 cm	0.2 cm
Basis of soft tissue contrast	Radiodensity	Biochemistry
Typical scanning time	10–20 minutes	40–60 minutes
Imaging plane	Transverse	Transverse, sagittal, coronal
Image streaking due to bone artifact	In certain areas	No

COMPARISON OF CT AND MRI—continued

	CT	MRI
Potential hazard with ferromagnetic objects	No	Yes
Cost	$200–$500	$700–$1000
Clinical indications	Intracranial calcifications, tumor margins, acute hemorrhage, agitated patient, limited time (acute head injury), contrast enhancement needed in some cases*	Demyelinating disease; pathology of: posterior fossa, apical areas, temporal areas, brain stem, spinal cord; can distinguish acute and chronic hemorrhage

*Intravenous (iv) contrast agent not necessary when looking for hemorrhage; it increases sensitivity of detecting mass lesions by only 5% and carries a significant risk in certain patient subgroups; iv contrast is contraindicated in patients with acute stroke.
Modified from Jaskiw GE, Andreasen NC, Weinberger DR: X-ray computed tomography and magnetic resonance imaging in psychiatry. Psychiatry Update 6:260–299, 1987.

DEXAMETHASONE SUPPRESSION TEST (DST)

I. *Procedure*: At 11:00 P.M. the patient should receive 1 mg of dexamethasone administered orally. On the following day, blood samples for measurement of plasma cortisols should be obtained at 8:00 A.M., 4:00 P.M., and 11:00 P.M. For many purposes, the 8:00 A.M. blood sample could be eliminated, because nearly all of the positive test results are detected on the 4:00 P.M. and 11:00 P.M. samples in combination. However, a low level of plasma cortisol in the 8:00 A.M. sample may verify that the dexamethasone was ingested.

II. *Interpretation of cortisol values*: The following general guidelines apply for the psychiatric DST

Plasma cortisol level (μg/dl)

0–4	Negative (suppression)
4–7	Borderline
7+	Positive (nonsuppression)

Physicians should consult their laboratories as to cortisol assay method and interpretation. The psychiatric DST measures low levels of cortisol that require precise and accurate standardization of laboratory assays.

Modified from the APA Task Force on Laboratory Tests in Psychiatry: The dexamethasone suppression test: an overview of its current status in psychiatry. Am J Psychiatry 144:1253–1262, 1987.

EXCLUSION CRITERIA FOR THE DEXAMETHASONE SUPPRESSION TEST

False-Positive Tests

Drugs:

Barbiturates	Meprobamate
Carbamazepine	Methaqualone
Glutethimide	Methyprylon
Estrogens (high dose)	Phenytoin

Alcohol or recent (3–4 weeks) withdrawal from alcohol

Endocrine abnormalities:
    Cushing's syndrome
    Diabetes mellitus (even if controlled)
    Hypercalcemia
    Pregnancy

Other medical conditions:
    Major medical disorder such as serious infection; recent major trauma or surgery; advanced renal or hepatic disease; uncontrolled cardiac failure or hypertension
    Fever, nausea, vomiting, dehydration
    Low body weight or recent weight loss
    Dementia

Suspected but not proven to interfere with DST:
    Brain tumor, temporal lobe disease, electroconvulsive therapy or grand mal seizure (on post-dexamethasone day), circadian phase advance
    Reserpine
    Hypothyroidism
    Recent withdrawal from antidepressants

EXCLUSION CRITERIA FOR THE DST—continued

False-Negative Tests

Drugs:
  Synthetic corticosteroids
  Isoniazid
  Methylphenidate

Endocrine abnormalities:
  Addison's disease
  Hypopituitarism
  Slow metabolism of dexamethasone

Suspected but not proven:
  Indomethacin
  High-dose benzodiazepine
  Tricyclic antidepressants
  L-Tryptophan

Modified from The APA Task Force on Laboratory Tests in Psychiatry: The dexametha-sone suppression test: an overview of its current status in psychiatry. Am J Psychiatry 144:1253–1262, 1987.

THERAPIES

PSYCHOPHARMACOLOGY

WHAT TO TELL
A PATIENT ABOUT A PRESCRIBED DRUG

1. Name of medicine (generic and trade)
2. Whether it is meant to treat the disease or to relieve symptoms, and the importance of taking it
3. How to tell if it is working, and what to do if it appears not to be working
4. When and how to take it—before or after meals
5. What to do if a dose is missed
6. How long to take it
7. Side effects that are important for the patient, and what to do about them
8. Possible effects on driving, on work, etc., and what precautions to take
9. Interactions with alcohol and other drugs
10. Anticipated cost
11. Degree of equivalence of generic preparations

Modified from Anonymous: What should we tell patients about their medicines? Drug Ther Bull 19:73–74, 1981.

TRADE NAME, GENERIC NAME,
AND DRUG CLASS

This table includes most clinically useful psychotropic agents. Also included are some drugs commonly used in psychiatry and a selection of commonly encountered analgesics, minor tranquilizers, and stimulants that may be potential drugs of abuse. Other pharmacologic agents are not included even though these agents may be relevant to psychiatric treatment. "Psychiatric use" refers to the most common use of these agents in psychiatry. Many drugs (e.g., diazepam) may have several other clinical uses.

TRADE NAME, GENERIC NAME, AND DRUG CLASS

Trade name	Generic name	Major psychiatric use (pharmacologic class)
Adapin	Doxepin	Antidepressant (tricyclic antidepressant)
Adipex	Phentermine	Anorectic (sympathomimetic amine)
Adipost	Phendimetrazine	Anorectic (amphetamine congener)
Akineton	Biperiden	Antiparkinsonian (anticholinergic)
Alurate	Aprobarbital	Minor tranquilizer (barbiturate)
Anafranil	Clomipramine	Treatment of obsessive-compulsive disorder (tricyclic antidepressant)
Antabuse	Disulfiram	Alcohol use deterrent (aldehyde dehydrogenase inhibitor)
Artane	Trihexyphenidyl	Antiparkinsonian (anticholinergic)
Asendin	Amoxapine	Antidepressant (cyclic antidepressant)
Atarax	Hydroxyzine	Minor tranquilizer (antihistamine)
Ativan	Lorazepam	Minor tranquilizer (benzodiazepine)
Aventyl	Nortriptyline	Antidepressant (tricyclic antidepressant)
B.A.C. no. 3	Butalbital, aspirin, caffeine, codeine	Analgesic (compound of barbiturate, nonsteroidal anti-inflammatory drug, stimulant, opiate)
Bancap HC	Acetaminophen, hydrocodone	Analgesic (compound of nonnarcotic and opiate analgesics)
Benadryl	Diphenhydramine	Minor tranquilizer (antihistamine)
Bellergal-S	Phenobarbital, ergotamine, belladonna alkaloids	Analgesic (compound of barbiturate, ergotamine, anticholinergic)
Biphetamine	Amphetamine with dextroamphetamine	Anorectic (amphetamine compound)
Bontril	Phendimetrazine	Anorectic (amphetamine congener)
Brevital	Methohexital injection	Minor tranquilizer (barbiturate)
BuSpar	Buspirone	Antianxiety agent
Butisol	Butabarbital	Minor tranquilizer (barbiturate)
Catapres	Clonidine	Antihypertensive, antimanic (α_2-adrenergic agonist)
Centrax	Prazepam	Minor tranquilizer (benzodiazepine)
Cibalith	Lithium citrate	Mood stabilizer (lithium salt)
Cogentin	Benztropine	Antiparkinsonian (antimuscarinic, antihistamine)
Compazine	Prochlorperazine	Antiemetic (phenothiazine)

Trade name	Generic name	Major psychiatric use (pharmacologic class)
Cylert	Pemoline	CNS stimulant (oxazolidine derivative)
Dalmane	Flurazepam	Minor tranquilizer (benzodiazepine)
Dantrium	Dantrolene sodium	Muscle relaxant
Darvocet	Propoxyphene, acetaminophen	Analgesic (compound of opiate agonist, acetaminophen)
Darvon	Propoxyphene	Analgesic (opiate agonist)
Demerol	Meperidine	Analgesic (opiate agonist)
Depakene	Valproic acid	Anticonvulsant (carboxylic acid)
Deprol	Meprobamate + benactyzine hydrochloride	Minor tranquilizer (compound of carbamate ester, anticholinergic)
Desoxyn	Methamphetamine	CNS stimulant (amphetamine)
Desyrel	Trazodone	Antidepressant (cyclic antidepressant)
Dexedrine	Dextroamphetamine	CNS stimulant (amphetamine)
Didrex	Benzphetamine	CNS stimulant (amphetamine congener)
Dilantin	Phenytoin	Anticonvulsant (hydantoin)
Dilaudid	Dihydromorphinone	Analgesic (opiate agonist)
Dolacet	Hydrocodone, acetaminophen	Analgesic (compound of opiate agonist, acetaminophen)
Dolene	Propoxyphene	Analgesic (opiate agonist)
Dolophine	Methadone	Analgesic (opiate agonist)
Donnatal	Phenobarbital, hyoscyamine, atropine, scopolamine	Antispasmodic (compound of barbiturate, antimuscarinic agents)
Doriden	Glutethimide	Hypnotic (piperidine derivative)
Duramorph	Morphine sulfate	Analgesic (opiate agonist)
Elavil	Amitriptyline	Antidepressant (tricyclic antidepressant)
Empirin	Aspirin	Analgesic (nonsteroidal anti-inflammatory drug)
Endep	Amitriptyline	Antidepressant (tricyclic antidepressant)
Epitol	Carbamazepine	Anticonvulsant, mood stabilizer (iminostilbene derivative)
Equagesic	Aspirin, meprobamate	Analgesic, minor tranquilizer (compound of nonsteroidal anti-inflammatory drug, carbamate derivative)
Equanil	Meprobamate	Hypnotic (carbamate derivative)
Eskalith	Lithium carbonate	Mood stabilizer (lithium salt)

TRADE NAME, GENERIC NAME, AND DRUG CLASS—continued

Trade name	Generic name	Major psychiatric use (pharmacologic class)
Etrafon	Perphenazine, amitriptyline	Major tranquilizer (compound of phenothiazine and tricyclic antidepressant)
Fastin	Phentermine	Anorectic (amphetamine congener)
Fiorinal	Aspirin, butalbital, caffeine	Analgesic (compound of nonsteroidal anti-inflammatory drug, barbiturate, and stimulant)
Halcion	Triazolam	Hypnotic (benzodiazepine)
Haldol	Haloperidol	Major tranquilizer (butyrophenone)
Inapsine	Droperidol	Major tranquilizer (butyrophenone)
Inderal	Propranolol	Antihypertensive (β-blocker)
Innovar	Fentanyl, droperidol	Major tranquilizer (compound of opiate agonist, butyrophenone)
Janimine	Imipramine	Antidepressant (tricyclic antidepressant)
Kemadrin	Procyclidine	Antiparkinsonian (anticholinergic)
Klonopin	Clonazepam	Minor tranquilizer (benzodiazepine)
Levo-Dromoran	Levorphanol tartrate	Analgesic (opiate agonist)
Levothroid	Levothyroxine	Thyroid hormone
Librax	Chlordiazepoxide, clidinium bromide	Minor tranquilizer (compound of benzodiazepine, anticholinergic)
Libritabs	Chlordiazepoxide	Minor tranquilizer (benzodiazepine)
Librium	Chlordiazepoxide	Minor tranquilizer (benzodiazepine)
Limbitrol	Chlordiazepoxide, amitriptyline	Psychoactive compound (benzodiazepine, tricyclic antidepressant)
Lithane	Lithium carbonate	Mood stabilizer (lithium salt)
Lithobid	Lithium carbonate	Mood stabilizer (lithium salt)
Lomotil	Diphenoxylate, atropine	Antispasmodic (compound of opiate agonist, antimuscarinic)
Lotusate	Talbutal	Minor tranquilizer (barbiturate)
Loxitane	Loxapine	Major tranquilizer (tricyclic dibenzoxapine)
Ludiomil	Maprotiline	Antidepressant (tetracyclic antidepressant)
Marplan	Isocarboxazid	Antidepressant (monoamine oxidase inhibitor)
Mazanor	Mazindol	Anorectic (isoindole)
Mebaral	Mephobarbital	Minor tranquilizer (barbiturate)
Melfiat	Phendimetrazine	Anorectic (amphetamine congener)

Trade name	Generic name	Major psychiatric use (pharmacologic class)
Mellaril	Thioridazine	Major tranquilizer (phenothiazine)
Menrium	Chlordiazepoxide, estrogens	Psychoactive compound (benzodiazepine, estrogens)
Mepergan	Promethazine, meperidine	Analgesic (compound of phenothiazine, opiate agonist)
Meprospan	Meprobamate, extended release form	Minor tranquilizer (carbamate derivative)
Miltown	Meprobamate	Minor tranquilizer (carbamate derivative)
Moban	Molindone	Major tranquilizer (dihydroindolone derivative)
Mysoline	Primidone	Anticonvulsant (barbiturate analogue)
Narcan	Naloxone	Opiate inhibitor (opiate antagonist)
Nardil	Phenelzine	Antidepressant (monoamine oxidase inhibitor)
Navane	Thiothixene	Major tranquilizer (thioxanthine)
Nembutal	Pentobarbital	Minor tranquilizer (barbiturate)
No Doz	Caffeine	CNS stimulant (xanthine derivative)
Noludar	Methyprylon	Hypnotic (piperidine derivative)
Norflex	Orphenadrine	Antiparkinsonian (anticholinergic)
Norpramin	Desipramine	Antidepressant (tricyclic antidepressant)
Nubain	Nalbuphine	Analgesic (partial opiate agonist)
Numorphan	Oxymorphone	Analgesic (opiate agonist)
Orap	Pimozide	Anti-Tourette's syndrome agent (diphenylbutyl piperidine)
Pamelor	Nortriptyline	Antidepressant (tricyclic antidepressant)
Parafon Forte	Chlorzoxazone, acetaminophen	Analgesic (compound of muscle relaxant, acetaminophen)
Parnate	Tranylcypromine	Antidepressant (monoamine oxidase inhibitor)
Pavulon	Pancuronium bromide	Neuromuscular blocking agent
Percocet	Oxycodone, acetaminophen	Analgesic (compound of opiate agonist, acetaminophen)
Percodan	Oxycodone, aspirin	Analgesic (compound of opiate agonist, nonsteroidal anti-inflammatory drug)
Percogesic	Phenyltoloxamine, acetaminophen	Analgesic (compound of opiate agonist, acetaminophen)
Periactin	Cyproheptadine	Antiparkinsonian (antihistamine, antiserotonin)
Permitil	Fluphenazine	Major tranquilizer (phenothiazine)

TRADE NAME, GENERIC NAME, AND DRUG CLASS—continued

Trade name	Generic name	Major psychiatric use (pharmacologic class)
Pertofrane	Desipramine	Antidepressant (tricyclic antidepressant)
Phenaphen	Acetaminophen; some have codeine	Analgesic compound
Phenergan	Promethazine	Antiemetic, minor tranquilizer (antihistamine, phenothiazine derivative)
Phenergan-D	Promethazine, pseudoephedrine	Decongestant (antihistamine, sympathomimetic)
Placidyl	Ethchlorvynol	Hypnotic (tertiary carbinol)
Plegine	Phendimetrazine	Anorectic (amphetamine congener)
PMB	Meprobamate, estrogens	Psychoactive compound (carbamate derivative, estrogens)
Pondimin	Fenfluramine	Anorectic (amphetamine congener)
Prelu-2	Phendimetrazine	Anorectic (amphetamine congener)
Preludin	Phenmetrazine	Anorectic (amphetamine congener)
Prolixin	Fluphenazine	Major tranquilizer (phenothiazine)
Prozac	Fluoxetine	Antidepressant (dibenzene propanamine)
Restoril	Temazepam	Minor tranquilizer (benzodiazepine)
Ritalin	Methylphenidate	CNS stimulant (piperidine derivative)
Roxanol	Morphine sulfate	Analgesic (opiate agonist)
Roxicodone	Oxycodone	Analgesic (opiate agonist)
Roxiprin	Aspirin, oxycodone	Analgesic (compound of opiate agonist, nonsteroidal anti-inflammatory drug)
Sanorex	Mazindol	Anorectic (isoindole)
Seconal	Secobarbital	Minor tranquilizer (barbiturate)
Seldane	Terfenadine	Decongestant (antihistamine)
Serax	Oxazepam	Minor tranquilizer (benzodiazepine)
Serentil	Mesoridazine	Major tranquilizer (phenothiazine)
Sinequan	Doxepin	Antidepressant (tricyclic antidepressant)
Solfoton	Phenobarbital	Anticonvulsant (barbiturate)
Sparine	Promazine	Major tranquilizer (phenothiazine)
Stadol	Butorphanol	Analgesic (partial opiate agonist)
Stelazine	Trifluoperazine	Major tranquilizer (phenothiazine)
Sublimaze	Fentanyl	Analgesic (opiate agonist)
Sufenta	Sufentanil	Analgesic (opiate agonist)
Surmontil	Trimipramine	Antidepressant (tricyclic antidepressant)

Trade name	Generic name	Major psychiatric use (pharmacologic class)
Symmetrel	Amantadine	Antiparkinsonian, antiviral
Synalgos-DC	Aspirin, caffeine, dihydrocodeine	Analgesic (compound of nonsteroidal anti-inflammatory, stimulant, and opiate agonist)
Synthroid	Levothyroxine	Thyroid hormone
Talacen	Pentazocine, acetaminophen	Analgesic (compound of opiate agonist, acetaminophen)
Talwin	Pentazocine	Analgesic (opiate agonist)
Taractan	Chlorprothixene	Major tranquilizer (thioxanthine)
Tegretol	Carbamazepine	Anticonvulsant, mood stabilizer (iminostilbene derivative)
Tenuate	Diethylpropion	Anorectic (sympathomimetic amine)
Tepanil	Diethylpropion	Anorectic (sympathomimetic amine)
Thorazine	Chlorpromazine	Major tranquilizer (phenothiazine)
Tofranil	Imipramine	Antidepressant (tricyclic antidepressant)
Tranxene	Clorazepate	Minor tranquilizer (benzodiazepine)
Trexan	Naltrexone	Opiate inhibitor (opiate antagonist)
Triavil	Perphenazine, amitriptyline	Psychoactive compound (phenothiazine, tricyclic antidepressant)
Trilafon	Perphenazine	Major tranquilizer (phenothiazine)
Tylox	Oxycodone, acetaminophen	Analgesic (compound of opiate agonist, acetaminophen)
Valium	Diazepam	Minor tranquilizer (benzodiazepine)
Valmid	Ethinamate	Minor tranquilizer (urethane)
Valrelease	Diazepam, extended release	Minor tranquilizer (benzodiazepine)
Versed	Midazolam	Minor tranquilizer (benzodiazepine)
Vicodin	Hydrocodone, acetaminophen	Analgesic (compound of opiate agonist, acetaminophen)
Vistaril	Hydroxyzine	Minor tranquilizer (antihistamine)
Vivactil	Protriptyline	Antidepressant (tricyclic antidepressant)
Vivarin	Caffeine	CNS stimulant (xanthine)
Wehless	Phendimetrazine	Anorectic (amphetamine congener)
Wellbutrin	Bupropion	Antidepressant (aminoketone)
Wygesic	Propoxyphene, acetaminophen	Analgesic (compound of opiate agonist, acetaminophen)
Xanax	Alprazolam	Minor tranquilizer (benzodiazepine)
Zarontin	Ethosuximide	Anticonvulsant (succinamide)

THERAPEUTIC AGENTS

This table contains information about drugs commonly used for psychiatric treatment. We have attempted to include those agents that are normally part of psychiatric practice. Some rarely used drugs have been omitted. Some agents (e.g., dantrolene and naloxone) are included for rapid reference even though information given here is necessarily brief. A few drugs (e.g., glutethimide) are not recommended for use but are included because they may be encountered in psychiatric populations.

Drugs are listed alphabetically by their generic name in the first column of the table. The most commonly encountered trade name is also listed. Doses for common psychiatric uses are listed in the second column. Doses are specified as "start," "maintenance," and "maximum." "Start" refers to the initial dose of the drug. This dose is increased as tolerated to the "maintenance dose," that is, the dose generally required for therapeutic efficacy. "Maximum" is the highest dose generally recognized as safe and effective. In some clinical circumstances this may be exceeded with appropriate monitoring.

Listed doses are for psychiatric uses and oral administration unless otherwise specified. Some drugs, such as antiparkinsonian or antihypertensive agents, may have other uses for which a different dose range is required. Doses for geriatric patients must be substantially decreased for many agents, especially the benzodiazepines, antidepressants, lithium, and some antipsychotics. Pediatric doses for some commonly used drugs are listed in a separate table immediately following this section. This listing is indicated by a note in the second column of the table.

The form supplied is listed in the third column for each drug. Information regarding the route of administration and parenteral dose is listed for some agents.

The fourth column lists the pharmacologic class of the agent and any features unique to its administration. Antidepressants, antiparkinsonians, antipsychotics, benzodiazepines, β-blockers, carbamazepine, disulfiram, lithium, and stimulants are discussed in more detail elsewhere in this manual. This is indicated by an asterisk following the general category of the drug. For other drugs, or for drugs in these categories with unique features, chief side effects or a short comment may be listed in this column.

This table has been prepared as a rapid reference and memory aid. Physicians are advised to consult standard reference works and package inserts for complete prescribing information for those agents with which they are unfamiliar.

Drug	Dose and route	Form supplied	Pharmacologic class/ unique features
Alprazolam (Xanax)	Maint: 0.25–0.5 mg q8h Max: 4 mg/day (some authors: 10 mg/day)	Tabs: 0.25/0.5/1 mg	Benzodiazepine*
Amantadine (Symmetrel)	For extrapyramidal symptoms: 100 mg q12h Recommended max: 300 mg/day	Caps: 100 mg Solution: 50 mg/5 ml	Antiparkinsonian,* antiviral Use with caution in patients with hepatic disease, renal disease, seizures, eczematoid dermatitis, or uncontrolled psychosis
Amitriptyline (Elavil, Endep)	Start: 50 mg/day as single bedtime dose or divided q12h Maint: 150–200 mg/day Max: 300 mg/day Children: See Pediatric Dose Table	Tabs: 10/25/50/75/100/150 mg Inj: 10 mg/ml	Antidepressant* Tricyclic Therapeutic plasma level: 80–250 ng/ml

THERAPEUTIC AGENTS—continued

Drug	Dose and route	Form supplied	Pharmacologic class/unique features
Amoxapine (Asendin)	Start: 50 mg q8–12h Maint: 200–300 mg/day (may be given as single bedtime dose) Max: 400–600 mg/day (close observation; use divided dose)	Tabs: 25/50/100/150 mg	Antidepressant* Dibenzoxapine class May rarely cause extrapyramidal symptoms or tardive dyskinesia Therapeutic plasma level: 200–600 ng/ml
Benztropine (Cogentin)	Max: 6 mg/day For extrapyramidal symptoms: 1–4 mg q12–24h orally For acute dystonic reaction: 1–2 mg im or iv Children: See Pediatric Dose Table	Tabs: 0.5/1/2 mg Inj: 1 mg/ml	Antiparkinsonian* Tertiary amine Antimuscarinic
Biperiden (Akineton)	For acute dystonic reaction: 2 mg im/iv q30 min to max 8 mg/day For extrapyramidal symptoms: 2 mg q8–24h orally	Tabs: 2 mg Inj: 5 mg/ml	Antiparkinsonian* Tertiary amine Antimuscarinic
Bupropion (Wellbutrin)	Start: 100 mg q12h Maint: 100 mg q8h Max: 450 mg/day	Tabs: 75/100 mg	Antidepressant* Aminoketone Agitation, dry mouth, insomnia, headache, nausea, constipation, tremor

			May have more risk of seizure than other antidepressants Single dose should not exceed 150 mg
Buspirone (BuSpar)	Start: 5 mg q8h Maint: 5–15 mg q8h Max: 60 mg/day	Tabs: 5/10 mg	Anxiolytic Dizziness, drowsiness, nausea, and headache are the most common side effects
Carbamazepine (Tegretol)	Start: 200 mg q12h Maint: 800–1,200 mg/day General max: 1,000–2,000 mg/day in adults but has been exceeded Children: See Pediatric Dose Table	Tabs: 100/200 mg Suspension: 100 mg/5 ml	Carbamazepine* Iminostilbene derivative Anticonvulsant, antimanic, useful in trigeminal neuralgia Hepatotoxicity, blood dyscrasias (including aplastic anemia), dermatologic disorders
Chlordiazepoxide (Libritabs, Librium)	Anxiolytic: 5–10 mg q6–8h orally, up to 20–25 mg q6–8h Dosage for treatment of sedative withdrawal may be much higher	Tabs: 5/10/25 mg Caps: 5/10/25 mg Inj: 100 mg/dry ampule	Benzodiazepine* Many active metabolites

THERAPEUTIC AGENTS—continued

Drug	Dose and route	Form supplied	Pharmacologic class/ unique features

Chlorpromazine (Thorazine)	Start: 25–75 mg q6–8h orally
	Maint: up to 400 mg/day
	Recommended max:
	  Outpatient: 800 mg/day
	  Inpatient: 2,000 mg/day
	Acute Sed: 25 mg im, may be re- peated hourly and increased over days to max 400 mg q4–6h in severe cases
	Children: See Pediatric Dose Table
		Extended release caps: 30/75/150/200/300 mg
		Tabs: 10/25/50/100/200 mg
		Solution: 10 mg/5 ml
		Concentrate: 30 mg/ml, 100 mg/ml
		Inj: 25 mg/ml
		Suppository: 25/100 mg
			Antipsychotic*
			Phenothiazine
			Ocular changes at high doses
			Nonspecific Q- and T-wave changes on electrocardiogram
			Hypotension

Chlorprothixene (Taractan)	Start: 10–50 mg q6–8h orally Max: 600 mg/day orally im dose: 25–50 mg up to 3 or 4 doses/24 h then change to oral dose	Tabs: 10/25/50/100 mg Concentrate: 100 mg/5 ml Inj: 12.5 mg/ml	Antipsychotic* Thioxanthine
Clonazepam (Klonopin)	Start: 0.5 mg q8h orally Max: 20 mg/day	Tabs: 0.5/1/2 mg	Benzodiazepine* Anticonvulsant
Clonidine (Catapres)	For detoxification of opiates: test dose 0.005–0.006 mg/kg orally; if patient responds, give 0.017 mg/kg/day divided into 3 or 4 doses per day for 10 days; usual dose = 0.3–1.2 mg/day	Tabs: 0.1/0.2/0.3 mg Transdermal patch: 0.1/0.2/ 0.3 mg per 24 h for 1 week	Imidazoline derivative Antihypertensive agent α_2-Adrenergic agonist Use with caution in patient with vascular or cardiac disease

Drug	Dosage	Preparations	Notes
Clorazepate (Tranxene)	For Tourette's in children: See Pediatric Dose Table	Tabs: 3.75/7.5/15 mg; Extended release tabs: 11.25/22.5 mg	Benzodiazepine* Active metabolites May be used in narcotic withdrawal May potentiate depression Can cause seizures and A-V block in acute overdose
Dantrolene sodium (Dantrium)	Neuroleptic malignant syndrome: 1 mg/kg iv repeated to max 10 mg/kg/dose; may repeat dose if symptoms recur; monitor closely	Caps: 25/50/100 mg; Inj: 20 mg with 3,000 mg mannitol in dry vial	Hydantoin-derived muscle relaxant Can cause hepatitis in long-term use
Desipramine (Norpramin, Pertofrane)	Start: 50 mg/day as single bedtime dose; Maint: 75–200 mg/day; Max: 300 mg/day	Tabs: 10/25/50/75/100/150 mg; Caps: 25/50 mg	Antidepressant* Tricyclic Therapeutic plasma level: 125–300 ng/ml
Dextro-amphetamine (Dexedrine)	Narcolepsy: 5–60 mg/day divided into 1–3 daily doses given early in day; For attention-deficit hyperactivity disorder: 5–10 mg 2 or 3 times daily; Max: 60 mg/day; Children: See Pediatric Dose Table	Tabs: 5/10/15 mg; Caps: 15 mg; Time-release caps: 5/10/15 mg; Elixir: 5 mg/5 ml	Stimulant* Amphetamine
Diazepam (Valium, Valrelease)	Anxiolytic dose: 2–10 mg q6–12h; Children: See Pediatric Dose Table	Tabs: 2/5/10 mg; Extended release caps: 15 mg; Inj: 5 mg/ml	Benzodiazepine* Active metabolites Anticonvulsant, muscle relaxant

THERAPEUTIC AGENTS—continued

Drug	Dose and route	Form supplied	Pharmacologic class/unique features
Diphenhydramine (Benadryl)	Oral: 25–50 mg q6–8h im or iv: 10–50 mg/dose Max: 400 mg/day im or iv Children: See Pediatric Dose Table	Tabs: 25/50 mg Caps: 25/50 mg Elixir: 12.5 mg/5 ml Solution: 12.5 mg/5 ml, 13.3 mg/5 ml Inj: 10 mg/ml, 50 mg/ml	Antihistamine May be used as sedative, hypnotic, for extrapyramidal symptoms, acute dystonic reactions, allergic reactions
Disulfiram (Antabuse)	Start: 250–500 mg as single A.M. dose Maint: 125–500 mg daily Max: 500 mg daily	Tabs: 250/500 mg	Aldehyde dehydrogenase inhibitor* Avoid alcohol, including over-the-counter preparations Hypersensitivity hepatitis and blood dyscrasias reported Avoid concomitant use of phenytoin
Doxepin (Adapin, Sinequan)	Start: 50–75 mg/day as single bedtime dose Maint: 75–150 mg/day Max: 300 mg/day	Caps: 10/25/50/75/100/150 mg Concentrate: 10 mg/ml	Antidepressant* Tricyclic, dibenzoxepin class Therapeutic plasma level: 150–250 ng/ml Solution inactivated by carbonated beverage
Ethchlorvynol (Placidyl)	Hypnotic: 500 mg–1 g at bedtime (500 mg is usual dose)	Caps: 200/500/750 mg	CNS depressant Avoid use for more than 1 week

Drug	Dosage	Preparations	Comments
			High potential for abuse; severe withdrawal syndrome Still in use, but not recommended
Fluoxetine (Prozac)	Start: 20 mg as single A.M. dose Maint: 20–80 mg/day Max: 80 mg/day	Caps: 20 mg	Antidepressant,* selective serotonin uptake blocker Benzene propanamine Nervousness, headache, insomnia, nausea are most common side effects; facial edema Discontinue if rash appears
Flurazepam (Dalmane)	Hypnotic: 15–30 mg at bedtime	Caps: 15/30 mg	Benzodiazepine* Active metabolites
Fluphenazine (Prolixin, Permitil)	Start: 1–2.5 mg q6–8h orally Maint: 1–5 mg/day orally after initial response Max: 20–40 mg/day orally For hydrochloride, im dose approximately equal 1/3–1/2 oral dose; usual im dose 1.25 mg, may be repeated q6–8h Max im: 10 mg/day For decanoate and enanthate, 20 mg/day orally approximately equal to 25 mg im q3wk Usual maint: 25 mg q2wk im	Decanoate: Inj: 25 mg/ml Enanthate: Inj: 25 mg/ml Hydrochloride: Tabs: 1/2.5/5/10 mg Elixir: 2.5 mg/5 ml Concentrate: 5 mg/ml Inj: 2.5 mg/ml	Antipsychotic* Phenothiazine Depression may occur with decanoate and enanthate

THERAPEUTIC AGENTS—continued

Drug	Dose and route	Form supplied	Pharmacologic class/ unique features
Glutethimide (Doriden)	Hypnotic: 250–500 mg at bedtime Max: 1 g/day	Tabs: 250/500 mg	CNS depressant High potential for abuse Severe sedative withdrawal with seizures Still in use, but not recommended
Haloperidol (Haldol)	Start: 0.5–5 mg q8–12h orally Max: 100 mg/day Acute agitation: 2–10 mg im; may repeat hourly Children: See Pediatric Dose Table Decanoate: start, 10–15 times previous daily oral dose to a maximum of 100 mg q4wk given im; adjust to patient response	Tabs: 0.5/1/2/5/10/20 mg Concentrate: 2 mg/ml Inj: 5 mg/ml Decanoate: Inj: 50 mg/ml	Antipsychotic* Butyrophenone
Hydroxyzine (Atarax, Vistaril)	Pruritus: 25 mg q6–8h orally Sedation: 50–100 mg q6h orally or 50–100 mg/dose im Nausea: 25–100 mg/dose im Potentiate opioids: 25–100 mg/dose im Children: See Pediatric Dose Table	Hydrochloride: Tabs: 10/25/50/100 mg Solution: 10 mg/5 ml Inj: 25 mg/ml, 50 mg/ml Pamoate: Caps: 25/50/100 mg Suspension: 25 mg/5 ml	Antihistamine Anticholinergic (weak) May potentiate other sedative agents

Drug	Dosage	Preparations	Category / Notes
Imipramine (Tofranil, Janimine)	Start: 50 mg/day as single bedtime dose Maint: 50–300 mg/day as single bedtime dose or divided into 2 or 3 doses per day Children: See Pediatric Dose Table	Tabs: 10/25/50 mg Caps: 75/100/125/150 mg Inj: 25 mg/2 ml	Antidepressant* Tricyclic Therapeutic plasma level: 150–250 ng/ml
Isocarboxazid (Marplan)	Start: 30 mg/day as single daily dose or divided into 2 to 3 doses per day Maint: 10–30 mg/day Recommended max: 30 mg/day	Tabs: 10 mg	Antidepressant Monoamine oxidase inhibitor*
Levothyroxine (Synthroid, Levothroid)	Adult mild hypothyroidism: 25–50 µg; increase by 25–50 µg at intervals of 2–4 wk until desired result	Tabs: 25/50/75/100/112/125/150/175/200/300 µg Inj: 200/500 µg	L-Thyroxine (T4)
Lithium carbonate (Eskalith, Lithane, Lithobid)	Start: low estimate of required dose; adjust to therapeutic blood level Usual adult dose: 900–1,800 mg/day in divided doses Children: See Pediatric Dose Table	Tabs: 300 mg (= 8.12 mEq) Extended-release tabs: 300/450 mg Coated tabs: 300 mg Caps: 300 mg (= 8.12 mEq)	Lithium* Therapeutic blood level initial: 0.8–1.3 mEq/L Therapeutic blood level maint: 0.5–0.8 mEq/L Toxic blood level: >1.5 mEq/L
Lithium citrate (Cibalith)	Same dosage as lithium carbonate	Oral solution: 8 mEq/5 ml	Fewer gastrointestinal side effects in some patients

THERAPEUTIC AGENTS—continued

Drug	Dose and route	Form supplied	Pharmacologic class/unique features
Lorazepam (Ativan)	Anxiolytic: 1–2 mg q8–12h Hypnotic: 2–4 mg at bedtime Recommended max: 10 mg/day in divided doses	Tabs: 0.5/1/2 mg Inj: 2 mg/ml, 4 mg/ml	Benzodiazepine* No metabolites Use injection with caution May cause severe arteriospasm if given ia
Loxapine (Loxitane)	Start: 10 mg orally q12h Maint: 50–100 mg/day divided q6–12h Max: 250 mg/day orally im dose: 12.5–50 mg q4–6h usually; q12h in some patients	Caps: 5/10/25/50 mg Concentrate: 25 mg/ml Inj: 50 mg/ml	Antipsychotic* Tricyclic dibenzoxapine Dermatitis, seizures Do not give iv Dilute oral solution prior to use Amoxapine is a metabolite
Maprotiline (Ludiomil)	Start: 50 mg/day as single bedtime dose Maint: 100–150 mg/day Max: 225 mg/day	Tabs: 25/50/75 mg	Antidepressant* Tetracyclic Associated with higher incidence of seizures than other cyclic antidepressants
Meprobamate (Equanil, Miltown)	Anxiolytic: 200–400 mg q6–12h Hypnotic: 800 mg at bedtime Max: 2,400 mg/day	Tabs: 200/400/600 mg	CNS depressant High potential for abuse, severe withdrawal Teratogenic Still in use, but not recommended

Drug	Dosage	Formulations	Class
Mesoridazine (Serentil)	Start: 25 mg q8h orally Maint: 100–400 mg/day orally im: 25 mg, may be repeated q30–60 min Max: 200 mg/day im	Tabs: 10/25/50/100 mg Concentrate: 25 mg/ml Inj: 25 mg/ml	Antipsychotic* Phenothiazine
Methadone (Dolophine)	Usual dose: 15–20 mg orally to acutely suppress symptoms of opiate withdrawal See section on narcotic withdrawal for detoxification schedule Usual starting dose for opiate maintenance: 20–40 mg/day as single daily dose Recommended max for maintenance: 40–100 mg/day	Tabs: 5/10 mg Dispersible tabs: 40 mg Solution: 5 mg/5 ml, 10 mg/5 ml, 10 mg/ml Inj: 10 mg/ml	Synthetic diphenylheptane-derivative opiate agonist Duration of action for analgesia: 4–6 h; extends to 22–48 h in patients on methadone maintenance for suppression of opiate withdrawal syndrome
Methamphetamine (Desoxyn)	Starting dose for attention-deficit hyperactivity disorder: 5 mg 1 to 3 times daily Usual effective dose: 20–25 mg/day Max: 40 mg/day	Tabs: 5 mg Extended-release tabs: 5/10/15 mg	Stimulant* Amphetamine
Methylphenidate (Ritalin)	Adult: 10 mg 2 or 3 times daily, early in day Maint: 10–60 mg/day Max: 60 mg/day Children: See Pediatric Dose Table	Tabs: 5/10/20 mg Extended-release tabs: 20 mg	Stimulant*

THERAPEUTIC AGENTS—continued

Drug	Dose and route	Form supplied	Pharmacologic class/ unique features
Midazolam (Versed)	Sedation: 0.035 mg/kg im or slow iv 1–2.5 mg/kg Max: 0.1–0.3 mg/kg	Inj: 1 mg/ml, 5 mg/ml	Benzodiazepine* Primarily for anesthesia or pre- or postoperative sedation Do not give iv if goal is sedated but awake patient
Molindone (Moban)	Start: 5–20 mg q6–8h Increase over 3–4 days to 100 mg/day Maint: 5–25 mg q6–8h Max: 225 mg/day	Tabs: 5/10/25/50/100 mg Concentrate: 20 mg/ml	Antipsychotic* Dihydroindolone derivative
Naloxone (Narcan)	Acute reversal of opiate toxicity: initial, 0.4–2 mg iv; repeat every 2–3 min if needed to max of 10 mg If no response after 10 mg, consider other clinical syndromes Children: See Pediatric Dose Table	Inj: 0.02 mg/ml, 0.4 mg/ml, 1 mg/ml	Semisynthetic opiate antagonist Onset of action: 1–2 min after iv injection, 2–5 min after sc or im injection Duration of action: 45 min Monitor patient after response; repeated doses may be needed

Naltrexone (Trexan)	Maintenance after opiate withdrawal: 50 mg/day, 100 mg q48h, 150 mg q72h	Tabs: 50 mg	Synthetic opiate antagonist Opiate antagonist activity onset 15–30 min; peaks at 12 h; declines after 24 h Use only in withdrawn patient (do naloxone challenge first) May cause dose-related hepatic injury
Nortriptyline (Pamelor)	Start: 25 mg/day as single bedtime dose Maint: 50–100 mg/day as single bedtime dose or 25–50 mg q8h Recommended max: 150 mg/day Children: See Pediatric Dose Table	Caps: 10/25/50/75 mg Solution: 10 mg/5 ml	Antidepressant* Tricyclic Therapeutic plasma level: 50–150 ng/ml Efficacy increases to a maximum and then decreases with increasing dose
Orphenadrine (Norflex, Disipal)	Parkinsonian symptoms: 100 mg q12h orally	Tab: 100 mg Inj: 30 mg/ml	Antiparkinsonian* Tertiary amine Antimuscarinic
Oxazepam (Serax)	Anxiolytic: 10–30 mg q6–8h	Tabs: 15 mg Caps: 10/15/30 mg	Benzodiazepine* No active metabolites
Pancuronium bromide (Pavulon)	Use only with adequate ventilatory support Dosage must be individualized Initial iv adult dose: 0.04–0.1 mg/kg	Inj: 1 mg/ml, 2 mg/ml	Synthetic, nondepolarizing neuromuscular blocking agent

THERAPEUTIC AGENTS—continued

Drug	Dose and route	Form supplied	Pharmacologic class/ unique features
Pemoline (Cylert)	Start: 37.5 mg/day as single A.M. dose Maint: 56–75 mg/day as single A.M. dose Max: 112.5 mg/day Children: See Pediatric Dose Table	Tabs: 18.75/37.5/75 mg Chewable tab: 37.5 mg	Stimulant* Oxazolidinone Produces abnormal liver enzymes; hepatic fatalities have been reported
Pentobarbital (Nembutal)	Hypnotic: 100–200 mg at bedtime orally Children: See Pediatric Dose Table	Caps: 50/100 mg Inj: 50 mg/ml Suppository: 30/60/120/200 mg	Barbiturate Short acting
Perphenazine (Trilafon)	Start: 4–6 mg q6-12h Maint: 8–64 mg/day as 2–16 mg q6–12h Usual im dose: 5 mg/dose; may be repeated after 6 h to total 15 mg/day outpatient or 30 mg/day inpatient Max: 24 mg/day outpatient; 64 mg/day inpatient	Tabs: 2/4/8/16 mg Concentrate: 16 mg/5 ml Inj: 5 mg/ml	Antipsychotic* Phenothiazine
Phenelzine (Nardil)	Start: 15 mg q8h Maint: 1 mg/kg/day as 15–30 mg q8h Max: 90 mg/day	Tabs: 15 mg	Monoamine oxidase inhibitor* Antidepressant

Drug	Dosage	Forms	Notes
Phenobarbital	Sedation: 30–120 mg/day as 10–40 mg q8–12h Hypnotic: 100–320 mg at bedtime orally Drug withdrawal: determine barbiturate dose to be replaced (see table of equivalents in section on sedative withdrawal) Children: See Pediatric Dose Table	Tabs: 8/16/32/65/100, 15/30/60 mg Caps: 16 mg Extended-release caps: 65 mg Elixir: 15 mg/5 ml, 20 mg/5 ml Inj: 30/60/65/130 mg/ml	Barbiturate Anticonvulsant Plasma level >50 µg/ml may produce coma Adjust dose to therapeutic serum level (20–40 µg/ml for adults) for anticonvulsant use
Phenytoin (Dilantin)	Start dose: 300 mg/day as 100 mg q8h Max: 600 mg/day Children: See Pediatric Dose Table	Chewable tabs: 50 mg Extended-release caps: 30/100 mg Caps: 30/100 mg Suspension: 30 mg/5 ml, 125 mg/5 ml Inj: 50 mg/ml	Anticonvulsant Adjust dose to obtain therapeutic serum level (10–20 µg/ml) Rashes common Teratogenic Precipitates in iv dextrose solution; must give in saline
Pimozide (Orap)	Start: 0.5 mg q12h Maint: <0.2 mg/kg/day or up to 10 mg/day, whichever is less Children: See Pediatric Dose Table	Tabs: 2 mg	Antipsychotic* Diphenylbutylpiperidine Electrocardiographic changes (prolonged Q-T)
Prazepam (Centrax)	Anxiolytic: 20–40 mg/day as single bedtime dose or divided q8–12h Hypnotic: 20 mg at bedtime	Tabs: 10 mg Caps: 5/10/20 mg	Benzodiazepine* Active metabolites

THERAPEUTIC AGENTS—continued

Drug	Dose and route	Form supplied	Pharmacologic class/unique features
Prochlorperazine (Compazine)	Start oral: 5–10 mg q6–8h Start im: 10–20 mg/dose; may be repeated after 2–4 h Max: 150 mg/day orally Children: See Pediatric Dose Table	Oral solution: 5 mg/5 ml Rectal suppository: 2.5/5/25 mg Edisylate: Solution: 5 mg/5 ml Inj: 5 mg/ml Maleate: Tabs: 5/10/25 mg Extended release caps: 10/15/30 mg	Antiemetic Phenothiazine Do not use if liver injury present Hepatotoxic
Procyclidine (Kemadrin)	Parkinsonism: 2.5–5 mg q8h For extrapyramidal symptoms: 2.5 mg q8h Max: 20 mg/day	Tabs: 5 mg	Antiparkinsonian* Tertiary amine Anticholinergic
Promethazine (Phenergan, Mepergan)	Sedation: 25–50 mg orally or im q4–6h Nausea: 12.5–25 mg rectally or im q4–6h Hypnotic: 12.5–50 mg at bedtime orally Children: See Pediatric Dose Table	Tabs: 12.5/25/50 mg Solution: 6.25 mg/5 ml, 25 mg/5 ml Inj: 25 mg/ml, 50 mg/ml (im only) Suppository: 12.5/25/50 mg	Sedative, antiemetic Phenothiazine derivative Antimuscarinic, antihistamine ia injection contraindicated sc injection contraindicated
Propranolol (Inderal)	Start dose: 20–40 mg q6–12h Increase over days to desired response	Tabs: 10/20/40/60/80 mg Extended-release caps: 60/80/120/160 mg	β-Adrenergic blocker* Mixed β₁ and β₂-blockade Withdraw over several days

	Max: 640 mg/day Children: See Pediatric Dose Table	Inj: 1 mg/ml	to avoid rebound hypertension
Protriptyline (Vivactil)	Start: 10–40 mg/day as 5–10 mg q6–12h Maint: 15–40 mg/day Max: 60 mg/day	Tabs: 5/10 mg	Antidepressant* Tricyclic Therapeutic plasma level: 70–260 ng/ml
Temazepam (Restoril)	Hypnotic: 15–30 mg at bedtime	Caps: 15/30 mg	Benzodiazepine* No active metabolites
Thioridazine (Mellaril)	Start: 25–100 mg q8h Max: 300 mg/day outpatient; 800 mg/day inpatient Children: See Pediatric Dose Table	Tabs: 10/15/25/50/100/150/ 200 mg Oral suspension: 25 mg/5 ml, 100 mg/5 ml Oral concentrate: 30 mg/ml, 100 mg/ml	Antipsychotic* Phenothiazine Retinopathy above 800 mg/ day May exacerbate cardiac arrhythmia
Thiothixene (Navane)	Start oral: 2–5 mg q8–12h Max: 60 mg/day orally im: 4 mg q6–12h Max: 30 mg/day im Children: See Pediatric Dose Table	Caps: 1/2/5/10/20 mg Oral concentrate: 5 mg/ml Inj: 2 mg/ml, 5 mg/ml	Antipsychotic* Thioxanthene
Tranylcypromine (Parnate)	Start: 10 mg q8h Maint: 30–60 mg/day Max: 60 mg/day	Tabs: 10 mg	Monoamine oxidase inhibitor* Contraindicated in persons >60 yr old; may cause cerebral sclerosis
Trazodone (Desyrel)	Start: 150 mg/day as 50 mg q8h Maint: 150–400 mg/day as single or divided dose Max: 400 mg/day outpatient; 600 mg/day inpatient	Tabs: 50/100/150 mg Breakable wafer: 300 mg	Antidepressant* Triazolopyridine Priapism Musculoskeletal pain

THERAPEUTIC AGENTS—continued

Drug	Dose and route	Form supplied	Pharmacologic class/ unique features
Triazolam (Halcion)	Hypnotic: 0.125–0.25 mg at bedtime Recommended max: 0.5 mg at bedtime	Tabs: 0.125/0.25 mg	Benzodiazepine*
Trifluoperazine (Stelazine)	Usual: 2–5 mg q12–24h orally Max: 20 mg/day outpatient; 40 mg/day inpatient im: 1–2 mg/dose up to 6–10 mg in 24 h Children: See Pediatric Dose Table	Tabs: 1/2/5/10 mg Oral solution: 10 mg/ml Inj: 2 mg/ml	Antipsychotic* Phenothiazine
Trihexyphenidyl (Artane)	For extrapyramidal symptoms: 5–15 mg/day divided into 1 to 3 doses	Tabs: 2/5 mg Extended-release caps: 5 mg Elixir: 2 mg/5 ml	Antiparkinsonian* Tertiary amine Antimuscarinic
Trimipramine (Surmontil)	Start: 50–100 mg/day as single dose at bedtime or 25 mg q8h Maint: 50–200 mg/day Max: 200 mg/day outpatient; 300 mg/day inpatient	Caps: 25/50/100 mg	Antidepressant* Tricyclic Therapeutic plasma level: 150–250 ng/ml

*Additional information about this class of agents is found later in this manual.
Caps = capsules; CNS = central nervous system; h = hour; ia = intra-arterial; im = intramuscular; inj = injection; iv = intravenous; maint = maintenance; max = maximum; q = every; sc = subcutaneous; tabs = tablets.

PEDIATRIC DOSAGE GUIDELINES FOR SELECTED PSYCHOTROPIC AGENTS

Drug doses in children must be carefully adjusted for the individual patient. Doses for most psychotropic drugs are less well established for children than for adults. Generally, prepubertal children ages 12 years or less require pediatric doses; older adolescents may require adult doses. Renal and hepatic clearance mechanisms function more efficiently in children than in adults. Use of blood-level monitoring is prudent to avoid toxicity and to ensure adequate dosing.

Drug	Dose	Recommended maximum
Amitriptyline*	Start: 50 mg/day divided q6–8h	150 mg/day (children are more sensitive to cardiovascular toxicity than are adults) Monitor EKG
Benztropine†	Maint: 0.5–6 mg/day orally, 1–2 mg/day im	6 mg/day
Carbamazepine‡	Start: 10 mg/kg/day divided q8–12h orally Maint: 10–30 mg/kg/day or 400–800 mg/day in children ages 6–12 yr	Ages 13–15 yr: 1 g/day Anticonvulsant therapeutic plasma level: 4–12 µg/ml (may need less than this for psychiatric uses)
Chlorpromazine	Start: 0.5 mg/kg q4–6h orally or 0.5 mg/kg q6–8h im Maint: 3–15 mg/kg/day, up to 50–200 mg/day, divided q6h	≤5 yr, weight <22.7 kg: 40 mg/day im 5–12 yr, weight 22–46 kg: 75 mg/day im

PEDIATRIC DOSAGE GUIDELINES FOR SELECTED PSYCHOTROPIC AGENTS—continued

Drug	Dose	Recommended maximum
Clonidine§	For Tourette's: Start: 0.05 mg/day (1 µg/kg/day), build up slowly (over 2–3 weeks) Maint: 0.1 mg q8h Must be tapered slowly	0.2 mg q8h (3–4 µg/kg/day)
Desipramine§	Adolescents: up to 150 mg/day	2.5 mg/kg/day
Dextroamphetamine†	Start: 3–5 yr: 2.5 mg/day orally; >5 yr: 5 mg/day orally in A.M. Maint: 0.5–0.75 mg/kg/day	1 mg/kg/day up to 40 mg/day
Diazepam	Anxiolytic doses (dose for other uses may vary): Start: 0.1–0.8 mg/kg/day divided q6–8h orally 0.1–0.3 mg/kg/dose im or slow iv Use large vein if given iv and have respiratory support available	15–30 mg/day orally ≤5 yr: 5 mg iv/dose >5 yr: 10 mg iv/dose
Diphenhydramine	Start: 5 mg/kg/day divided q6–8h orally Maint: 2–5 mg/kg/day Hypnotic: 1 mg/kg or 25–50 mg at bedtime Acute dystonic reaction: 25–50 mg im followed by 25–50 mg orally	300 mg/day

Drug	Dosage	Notes
Haloperidol[†]	Start: 0.05–0.15 mg/kg/day divided q8–12h in children 3–12 yr Maint: 0.1–0.5 mg/kg/day For Tourette's: 0.05–0.075 mg/kg/day divided q8–12h in children 3–12 yr (weight 15–40 kg)	3–12 yr: 6 mg/day im or orally
Hydroxyzine	2 mg/kg/day divided q6h orally 0.5–1.0 mg/kg/day im Sedative: 25–50 mg at bedtime	>6 yr: 100 mg/day <6 yr: 50 mg/day
Imipramine[‡]	Depression: Start: 0.5 mg/kg/day as single bedtime dose Maint: 3–4.5 mg/kg/day Enuresis: 0.3–2.5 mg/kg/day (25–50 mg 1 h prior to bedtime) Attention-deficit hyperactivity disorder: 0.3–2.5 mg/kg/day as single bedtime dose	FDA: 2.5 mg/kg/day Some authors: 4.5 mg/kg/day (children are more sensitive to cardiovascular toxicity than are adults) Monitor EKG
Lithium*	Start: 150 mg/day Maint: 150 mg/day and up (300–900 mg/day for children and adolescents)	Monitor blood levels closely; therapeutic blood level: 0.5–1.3 mEq/L
Methylphenidate[‡]	Start: 5 mg orally in A.M. and at midday Maint: 5–10 mg orally 2 or 3 times daily or 0.3–0.5 mg/kg/day in divided doses Administration in the evening may disrupt sleep	60 mg/day

PEDIATRIC DOSAGE GUIDELINES FOR SELECTED PSYCHOTROPIC AGENTS—continued

Drug	Dose	Recommended maximum
Naloxone	Start: 0.01 mg/kg/dose iv If no improvement, give 0.1 mg/kg/dose up to 0.4 mg total Monitor closely if patient responds; duration of action = 45 min. Repeat administration as needed	0.4 mg
Nortriptyline*	Adolescents: 30–50 mg/day	Monitor EKG
Pemoline‡	Start: 37.5 mg/day as single A.M. dose Increase weekly to effective dose, by 18.75 mg/day per week Maint: 37.5–112.5 mg/day (1.0–2.5 mg/kg/day)	112.5 mg/day
Pentobarbital	2–6 mg/kg/day divided q8h orally/im/rectally for acute sedation	Orally/im max: 100 mg/day or dose
Phenobarbital	Sedation: 2–3 mg/kg/dose orally/im/rectally, may be given q8h Anticonvulsant: 4–6 mg/kg/day divided q12h orally	Anticonvulsant therapeutic plasma level: 15–30 µg/ml
Phenytoin	4–8 mg/kg/day divided q8–12h orally or iv	Anticonvulsant therapeutic plasma level: 10–20 µg/ml

Pimozide	Tourette's: 0.2 mg/kg/day or from 1–10 mg/day (little information on use in children <12 yr)	0.2 mg/kg/day up to 10 mg/day total
Prochlorperazine//	0.4 mg/kg/day divided q6–8h orally/rectally for nausea 0.13 mg/kg im, initial dose, then change to orally or rectally	Age (yr) Dose (mg/day) 2–5 20 6–12 25 Avoid if symptoms suggest Reye's syndrome Do not use in pediatric surgery Relatively high incidence of extrapyramidal symptoms in children
Promethazine//	Nausea: 0.1–0.5 mg/kg/dose q4–6h im/orally/rectally Sedation: 0.5–1.0 mg/kg/dose q6h im	
Propranolol	≤35 kg: 10–20 mg q8h orally >35 kg: 20–40 mg q8h orally or 1–4 mg/kg/day divided q8–12h	16 mg/kg/day Adult max: 640 mg/day
Thioridazine//	Start: 0.5–3.0 mg/kg/day divided q6–12h Maint: 3–6 mg/kg/day (10–25 mg q8–12h)	≤12 yr: 3.0 mg/kg/day Adult max: 800 mg/day

PEDIATRIC DOSAGE GUIDELINES FOR SELECTED PSYCHOTROPIC AGENTS—continued

Drug	Dose	Recommended maximum
Thiothixene*	Adolescents: Use minimal adult dose: 6–15 mg/day divided q8–12h	60 mg/day
Trifluoperazine	Start: 1 mg q12–24h orally Increase gradually to control symptoms Dose in children <6 yr not established	15 mg/day

*Not recommended by FDA for children <12 yr.
†Not recommended by FDA for children <3 yr.
‡Not recommended by FDA for children <6 yr.
§Not recommended by FDA for use in children.
‖Not recommended by FDA for children <2 yr.

im = intramuscular; iv = intravenous; maint = maintenance; q = each/every.

See also:

Popper CW: Child and adolescent psychopharmacology, in Psychiatry, Vol. 2. Edited by Michels R, Cavenar J, Brodie K, et al. Philadelphia, PA, JB Lippincott, 1985, pp 1–23.

Rifkin A, Wortman R, Reardon G, et al: Psychotropic medication in adolescents: a review. J Clin Psychiatry 47:400–408, 1986.

Robson KS (ed): Manual of Clinical Child Psychiatry. Washington, DC, American Psychiatric Press, 1986.

USE OF THERAPEUTIC DRUG LEVEL MONITORING

Measurements of drug levels in blood or plasma have many uses in psychiatry, but they do not replace the use of clinical judgment. The following are some guidelines about the use of blood level measurements. For lithium and a few of the tricyclic antidepressants (amitriptyline, nortriptyline, imipramine, and desipramine), therapeutic blood levels have been clearly established. For other antidepressants, the neuroleptics, and the anticonvulsants when used for treatment of psychiatric disorders, blood levels are useful in some circumstances, but therapeutic levels have not been established with the same degree of certainty.

WHEN TO MEASURE BLOOD LEVELS OF PSYCHOTROPIC DRUGS

1. When patient fails to respond: inadequate dose or noncompliance
2. To monitor effective dosing of a potentially toxic agent (e.g., lithium) or treatment of patients with poor tolerance for side effects (e.g., elderly patients, medically ill, or children)
3. When toxicity is suspected
4. To document the level of a therapeutic dose for an individual patient, especially those patients requiring unusually high or low doses
5. To expedite rapid treatment of suicidal or hospitalized patients

PRINCIPLES OF DRUG MONITORING BY BLOOD LEVEL

1. Drug levels are most reliably measured as "trough" levels; just before the next dose, generally in the morning
2. Patients should be at a pharmacokinetically stable level; after at least five drug half-lives (generally, after five doses)
3. As with any laboratory test, results should be interpreted with the patient's clinical condition in mind

Therapeutic levels for antidepressants, lithium, and selected anticonvulsants are listed elsewhere in this manual in the Table of

Therapeutic Agents and also in the relevant section for that psychotropic agent.

See also:

Task Force on the Use of Laboratory Tests in Psychiatry: Tricyclic antidepressants—blood level measurements and clinical outcome: an APA Task Force Report. Am J Psychiatry 142:155–162, 1985.

Yesavage JA: Psychotropic blood levels: a guide to clinical response. J Clin Psychiatry 47 (suppl):16–19, 1986.

RELATIVE POTENTIAL OF PSYCHOTROPICS FOR LOWERING THE SEIZURE THRESHOLD

	Antipsychotics	Antidepressants	Other
High	Chlorpromazine	Maprotiline Amoxapine* Amitriptyline Imipramine Nortriptyline	
Moderate	Thiothixene Haloperidol†	Protriptyline	Lithium
Moderate to low	Perphenazine Trifluoperazine	Trimipramine Desipramine	
Low	Fluphenazine Thioridazine‡ Molindone	Doxepin‡	Meprobamate Glutethimide Methaqualone Ethchlorvynol
Anticonvulsant		MAOIs	Benzodiazepines Methylphenidate Dextroamphetamine
Unknown	Loxapine	Trazodone	

---

*Based on high incidence of seizures in overdose. See: Litovitz TL, Troutman WG: Amoxapine overdose: seizures and fatalities. JAMA 250:1069–1071, 1983.

†Haloperidol has been safer clinically than animal and in vitro studies indicate.

‡May be more epileptogenic at low doses.

Modified from Mendez MF, Cummings JL, Benson DF: Epilepsy: psychiatric aspects and use of psychotropics. Psychosomatics 25:883–894, 1984.

USE OF THE RECEPTOR AFFINITY TABLES

Most clinicians have learned to prescribe drugs by memorizing the side-effect profiles for each compound and by building familiarity through clinical applications of the drugs. Psychopharmacology can be especially confusing if approached in this manner, because many compounds have similar side-effect profiles that differ in intensity. For example, the tricyclic antidepressants and neuroleptics share anticholinergic properties, but some agents are more troublesome clinically than others.

A useful method for quickly determining the principal side effects and their relative intensities is the use of tables of receptor affinities. These tables reflect the propensity of a given compound to block a particular neurotransmitter receptor or uptake site. When pharmacologic in vitro binding studies are compared to in vivo assays of biologic activity, knowledge of the receptor affinities alone can be shown to predict the activity of the compound within that neurotransmitter system.

What follows are several tables related to this concept. The first is a list of key neurotransmitter systems and the physiologic variables affected by each. This is followed by separate tables for the dopaminergic, muscarinic, α_1-adrenergic, and histaminic receptors and their affinities for the neuroleptics and most antidepressants. A higher value for affinity represents greater potency in blockade of the receptor and increased likelihood of clinical effect. Although small numerical differences in these values may not be reflected clinically, differences in orders of magnitude almost certainly are. For example, amitriptyline has a potency (K_d) of 5.5 at the muscarinic acetylcholine receptor (responsible for most anticholinergic side effects), whereas desipramine has a value of 0.50 and trazodone of only 0.00031.

Finally, at the end of this section complete tables of the antidepressant and antipsychotic agents and their affinities in human brain are presented. The organization of these final tables is by drug listing, rather than in the order of receptor affinities. All of the receptor affinities are listed again, along with others (e.g., serotonin) that are relevant in certain clinical circumstances. Readers who are familiar with the use of receptor affinities to predict side effects of psychopharmacologic agents will probably find these tables faster to use.

Two complete tables are included for the neuroleptic agents. The first presents the receptor affinities measured in vitro. The second presents the same data adjusted to include the affinity of the compound for the dopamine subtype 2 (D_2) receptor, which is believed to be responsible for the antipsychotic properties of these compounds. In this way, the relative potency of the neuroleptics for other neurotransmitter systems can be compared, having allowed for the fact that some agents are high potency (e.g., haloperidol) and others are low potency (e.g., chlorpromazine) at the D_2 receptor. Only the adjusted data are presented in the summary tables.

One limitation of this method for selecting psychotropic agents is that it predicts actions of agents in the central nervous system only. Pharmacokinetic properties, such as absorption, distribution, metabolism, and protein binding also contribute to the intensity of the side-effect profile. However, while keeping this in mind, the clinician who becomes familiar with the receptor affinity concept will find it a powerful tool in selecting and prescribing psychiatric drugs.

See also:

Pollack MH, Rosenbaum JF: Management of antidepressant-induced side effects: a practical guide for the clinician. J Clin Psychiatry 48:3–8, 1987.

Richelson E: Are receptor studies useful for clinical practice? J Clin Psychiatry 44:4–9, 1983.

PHARMACOLOGIC CONSEQUENCES OF RECEPTOR BINDING BY PSYCHOACTIVE AGENTS (SIDE EFFECTS ORGANIZED BY RECEPTOR BLOCKADE)

Property	Possible clinical consequences
Blockade of norepinephrine uptake at nerve endings	Alleviation of depression Tremors Tachycardia Erectile and ejaculatory dysfunction Blockade of the antihypertensive effects of guanethidine (Ismelin and Esimil) and guanadrel (Hylorel) Augmentation of pressor effects of sympathomimetic amines

Property	Possible clinical consequences
Blockade of serotonin uptake at nerve endings	Alleviation of depression Postural hypotension
Blockade of histamine H_1 receptors	Potentiation of central depressant drugs Sedation, drowsiness Weight gain Hypotension
Blockade of muscarinic receptors	Blurred vision Dry mouth Sinus tachycardia Constipation Urinary retention Memory dysfunction
Blockade of α_1-adrenergic receptors	Potentiation of the antihypertensive effect of prazosin (Minipress) Postural hypotension, dizziness Reflex tachycardia
Blockade of α_2-adrenergic receptors	Blockade of the antihypertensive effects of clonidine (Catapres), guanabenz (Wytensin), and α-methyldopa (Aldomet)
Blockade of dopamine D_2 receptors	Extrapyramidal movement disorders Endocrine changes (prolactin elevation)
Blockade of serotonin 5-HT_2 receptors	Ejaculatory dysfunction Hypotension Alleviation of migraine headaches

From Richelson E: Antidepressants: pharmacology and clinical use, in Treatments of Psychiatric Disorders. Edited by Karasu TB. Washington, DC, American Psychiatric Association, 1989, pp 1773–1787. By permission of the publisher.

DOPAMINE D_2 RECEPTOR

Blockade of the dopamine receptor is probably instrumental in the antipsychotic action of the neuroleptics. It is certainly involved in the development of extrapyramidal side effects of these drugs.

As a class, the antidepressants do not significantly block the dopamine D_2 receptor. Affinities range from 0.026 (trazodone) to 0.625 (amoxapine).

---

*Affinities of Neuroleptics for the Dopamine Receptor**

Thiothixene	222	Mesoridazine	5.3
Fluphenazine	125	Thioridazine	3.8
Perphenazine	71	Loxapine	1.4
Trifluoperazine	38	Molindone	0.83
Haloperidol	25	Clozapine	0.56
Prochlorperazine	14	Reference compound	
Chlorprothixene	13	Haloperidol	25
Chlorpromazine	5.3		

*Units: 10^7 x $1/K_d$, where K_d is the equilibrium dissociation constant expressed in molarity.

MUSCARINIC RECEPTOR

The muscarinic receptor is the subtype of cholinergic receptor most affected by psychotropic compounds. (The other cholinergic receptor is the nicotinic, which is found mainly in the peripheral nervous system.) Blockade of the muscarinic receptor results in dry mouth, constipation, blurred vision (through interference with accommodation), decreased sweating, memory difficulty, and urinary retention.

*Affinities of Antidepressants for the Muscarinic Receptor**

Amitriptyline	5.5	Desipramine	0.50
Protriptyline	4.0	Maprotiline	0.18
Trimipramine	1.7	Amoxapine	0.10
Doxepin	1.2	Fluoxetine	0.050
Imipramine	1.1	Bupropion	0.0021
Nortriptyline	0.67	Trazodone	0.00031

Affinities of Neuroleptics for the Muscarinic Receptor†

Clozapine	15	Perphenazine	0.00093
Thioridazine	1.4	Fluphenazine	0.00042
Mesoridazine	0.28	Molindone	0.00031
Chlorpromazine	0.27	Haloperidol	0.00017
Loxapine	0.16	Thiothixene	0.00016
Prochlorperazine	0.013	Reference compound	
Trifluoperazine	0.0039	Atropine	42

*Units: 10^7 x $1/K_d$, where K_d is the equilibrium dissociation constant expressed in molarity.

†Units: $\dfrac{\text{Neuroreceptor affinity (drug X)}}{\text{Dopamine } D_2 \text{ receptor affinity (drug X)}}$.

α_1-ADRENERGIC RECEPTOR

Blockade of the α_1-adrenergic receptor causes orthostatic hypotension through a central mechanism (or by peripheral vasodilatation), accompanied by dizziness and a reflex tachycardia. Blockade at this receptor potentiates the effect of the antihypertensive agent prazosin, which also acts through this receptor.

Affinities of Antidepressants for the α_1-Adrenergic Receptor*

Doxepin	4.2	Maprotiline	1.1
Trimipramine	4.2	Imipramine	1.1
Amitriptyline	3.7	Protriptyline	0.77
Trazodone	2.8	Desipramine	0.77
Amoxapine	2.0	Bupropion	0.022
Nortriptyline	1.7	Fluoxetine	0.017

Affinities of Neuroleptics for the α_1-Adrenergic Receptor†

Clozapine	20	Perphenazine	0.14
Mesoridazine	9.5	Trifluoperazine	0.11
Chlorpromazine	7.3	Fluphenazine	0.088
Thioridazine	5.2	Thiothixene	0.041
Loxapine	2.5	Reference compound	
Haloperidol	0.66	Phentolamine	6.7
Prochlorperazine	0.30		

---

*Units: $10^7 \times 1/K_d$, where K_d is the equilibrium dissociation constant expressed in molarity.

†Units: $\dfrac{\text{Neuroreceptor affinity (drug X)}}{\text{Dopamine } D_2 \text{ receptor affinity (drug X)}}$

HISTAMINE H_1 RECEPTOR

This receptor is believed responsible for the sedating effect of many compounds, in addition to more troublesome side effects such as weight gain, hypotension, and potentiation of other sedative-hypnotic compounds.

*Affinities of Antidepressants for the Histamine H_1 Receptor**

Doxepin	420	Amoxapine	4.0
Trimipramine	370	Protriptyline	4.0
Amitriptyline	91	Desipramine	0.91
Maprotiline	50	Trazodone	0.29
Nortriptyline	10	Fluoxetine	0.016
Imipramine	9.1	Bupropion	0.015

Affinities of Neuroleptics for the Histamine H_1 Receptor†

Clozapine	64	Thiothixene	0.075
Loxapine	14	Trifluoperazine	0.042
Mesoridazine	10	Fluphenazine	0.038
Chlorpromazine	2.1	Haloperidol	0.0021
Thioridazine	1.6	Molindone	0.00097
Prochlorperazine	0.37	Reference compound	
Perphenazine	0.18	Diphenhydramine	7.1

*Units: $10^7 \times 1/K_d$, where K_d is the equilibrium dissociation constant expressed in molarity.

†Units: $\dfrac{\text{Neuroreceptor affinity (drug X)}}{\text{Dopamine } D_2 \text{ receptor affinity (drug X)}}$.

ANTIDEPRESSANT POTENCIES* FOR BLOCKING UPTAKE OF NOREPINEPHRINE (NE) AND SEROTONIN (5-HT) AND AFFINITIES† FOR SOME NEUROTRANSMITTER RECEPTORS

Drug (generic and trade names)	Uptake blockade*‡			Receptor blockade†§					
			Ratio	Histamine		α-Adrenergic		Dopamine	Serotonin
	NE	5-HT	NE/5-HT	H_1	Muscarinic	α_1	α_2	D_2	$5\text{-}HT_2$
Tricyclic: tertiary amines									
Amitriptyline (Elavil, Endep)	4.2	1.5	2.8	91	5.5	3.7	0.11	0.10	3.4
Doxepin (Adapin, Sinequan)	5.3	0.36	15	420	1.2	4.2	0.091	0.042	4.0
Imipramine (Tofranil, SK-Pramine)	7.7	2.4	3.2	9.1	1.1	1.1	0.031	0.050	1.2
Trimipramine (Surmontil)	0.20	0.040	5.0	370	1.7	4.2	0.15	0.56	3.1
Tricyclic: secondary amines									
Desipramine (Norpramin, Pertofrane)	110	0.29	380	0.91	0.50	0.77	0.014	0.030	0.36
Nortriptyline (Pamelor)	25	0.38	66	10	0.67	1.7	0.040	0.83	2.3
Protriptyline (Vivactil)	100	0.36	280	4.0	4.0	0.77	0.015	0.43	1.4
Dibenzoxazepine									
Amoxapine (Asendin)	23	0.21	110	4.0	0.10	2.0	0.038	0.625	170
Tetracyclic									
Maprotiline (Ludiomil)	14	0.030	470	50	0.18	1.1	0.011	0.28	0.83
Triazolopyridine									
Trazodone (Desyrel)	0.020	0.53	0.038	0.29	0.00031	2.8	0.20	0.026	14

Benzenepropanamine								
Fluoxetine (Prozac)	0.36	8.3	0.043	0.016	0.050	0.017	0.0077	0.36	0.48
Propiophenone								
Bupropion (Wellbutrin)	0.043	0.0064	6.7	0.015	0.0021	0.022	0.0012	0.00048	0.0011
Reference compounds								
d-Amphetamine (Dexedrine)	2.0								
Diphenhydramine (Benadryl)			7.1						
Atropine					42				
Phentolamine (Regitine)						6.7	2.3		
Haloperidol (Haldol)								25	
Methysergide (Sansert)									15

*$10^7 \times 1/K_i$, where K_i is the inhibitor constant in molarity.

†$10^7 \times 1/K_d$, where K_d is the equilibrium dissociation constant in molarity.

‡Data modified from Richelson E, Pfenning M: Blockade by antidepressants and related compounds of biogenic amine uptake into rat brain synaptosomes: most antidepressants selectively block norepinephrine uptake. Eur J Pharmacol 104:277–286, 1984.

§Data modified from Richelson E, Nelson A: Antagonism by antidepressants of neurotransmitter receptors of normal human brain in vitro. J Pharmacol Exp Ther 230:94–102, 1984. Wander TJ, Nelson A, Okazaki H, et al: Antagonism by antidepressants of serotonin S_1 and S_2 receptors of normal human brain in vitro. Eur J Pharmacol 132:115–121, 1986.

From Richelson E: Antidepressants: pharmacology and clinical use, in Treatments of Psychiatric Disorders. Edited by Karasu TB. Washington, DC, American Psychiatric Association, 1989, pp 1773–1787. By permission of the publisher.

AFFINITIES* OF SOME ANTIPSYCHOTIC AGENTS FOR SEVERAL NEUROTRANSMITTER RECEPTORS

Antipsychotic agent (trade name)	Receptor					
	Dopamine D_2	Histamine H_1	Adrenergic			Muscarinic
			α_1	α_2		
Chlorpromazine (Thorazine)	5.3	11	38	0.13		1.4
Chlorprothixene (Taractan)	13	...	...	...		...
Clozapine (Clozaril)	0.56	36	11	0.62		8.3
Fluphenazine (Permitil, Prolixin)	125	4.8	11	0.064		0.053
Haloperidol (Haldol)	25	0.053	16	0.026		0.0042
Loxapine (Loxitane)	1.4	20	3.6	0.042		0.22
Mesoridazine (Serentil)	5.3	55	50	0.062		1.4
Molindone (Moban)	0.83	0.00081	0.040	0.16		0.00026
Perphenazine (Trilafon)	71	12	10	0.20		0.067
Prochlorperazine (Compazine)	14	5.3	4.2	0.059		0.18
Thioridazine (Mellaril)	3.8	6.2	20	0.12		5.6
Thiothixene (Navane)	222	17	9.1	0.50		0.034
Trifluoperazine (Stelazine)	38	1.6	4.2	0.038		0.15

*$10^{-7} \times 1/K_d$, where K_d is the equilibrium dissociation constant in molarity.

Modified from Richelson E, Nelson A: Antagonism by neuroleptics of neurotransmitter receptors of normal human brain in vitro. Eur J Pharmacol 103:197–204, 1984.

See also: Black JL, Richelson E: Antipsychotic agents: prediction of side-effect profiles based on neuroreceptor data derived from human brain tissue. Mayo Clin Proc 62:369–372, 1987.

NEURORECEPTOR AFFINITIES FOR SEVERAL ANTIPSYCHOTIC AGENTS STANDARDIZED TO EQUIVALENT DOPAMINE D₂ RECEPTOR BLOCKADE

This is a comparison of relative drug potencies at various receptors when the patient receives a dose of drug sufficient to cause equivalent dopamine receptor blockade.

	Receptor			
	Histamine	Adrenergic		
Antipsychotic agent	H_1	α_1	α_2	Muscarinic
Chlorpromazine	2.1	7.3	0.025	0.27
Clozapine	64	20	1.1	15
Fluphenazine	0.038	0.088	0.00051	0.00042
Haloperidol	0.0021	0.66	0.0010	0.00017
Loxapine	14	2.5	0.029	0.16
Mesoridazine	10	9.5	0.012	0.28
Molindone	0.00097	0.048	0.19	0.00031
Perphenazine	0.18	0.14	0.0027	0.00093
Prochlorperazine	0.37	0.30	0.0041	0.013
Thioridazine	1.6	5.2	0.032	1.4
Thiothixene	0.075	0.041	0.0022	0.00016
Trifluoperazine	0.042	0.11	0.010	0.0039

Standardized neuroreceptor affinity $= \dfrac{\text{Neuroreceptor affinity (drug X)}}{\text{Dopamine } D_2 \text{ receptor affinity (drug X)}}$.

A higher numerical value indicates greater blockade of a given receptor when a dopamine receptor-blocking dose is given.

From Black JL, Richelson E: Antipsychotic drugs: prediction of side-effect profiles based on neuroreceptor data derived from human brain tissue. Mayo Clin Proc 62:369–372, 1987. By permission of Mayo Foundation.

ANTIPSYCHOTIC DRUGS

POTENCY AND RANGE OF ORAL DOSE OF NEUROLEPTICS

Antipsychotic agent: generic name (trade name)	Approximate amount (mg) of drug needed to equal 100 mg of chlorpromazine	Range of daily oral dose (mg)
Aliphatic		
Chlorpromazine (Thorazine)	100	25–2,000
Piperazine		
Fluphenazine (Permitil, Prolixin)	2	1–40
Perphenazine (Trilafon)	10	4–64
Prochlorperazine (Compazine)	15	15–150
Trifluoperazine (Stelazine)	5	2–40
Piperidine		
Mesoridazine (Serentil)	50	75–400
Thioridazine (Mellaril)	100	75–800
Butyrophenone		
Haloperidol (Haldol)	2	1–100
Thioxanthene		
Chlorprothixene (Taractan)	100	30–600
Thiothixene (Navane)	4	6–60
Dihydroindolone		
Molindone (Moban)	10	15–225
Dibenzoxazepine		
Loxapine (Loxitane)	10	10–250

Modified from Black JL, Richelson E, Richardson JW: Antipsychotic agents: a clinical update. Mayo Clin Proc 60:777–789, 1985.
See also: Mason AS, Granacher RP: Clinical Handbook of Antipsychotic Drug Therapy. New York, Brunner/Mazel, 1980.

SIDE EFFECTS OF ANTIPSYCHOTIC DRUGS

Early Onset and Commonly Encountered

Antimuscarinic effects

Blurred vision	Constipation
Urinary retention	Decreased sweating
Dry mouth	Memory difficulty

Antihistaminic effects
Sedation
Drowsiness
Potentiation of central nervous system depressants

Anti-α-adrenergic effects
Dizziness, lightheadedness, postural hypotension

Variable Onset (dopaminergic effects)
Acute dyskinesia, muscle spasms
Akathisia
Parkinsonism
Neuroleptic malignant syndrome*
Hyperprolactinemia, galactorrhea

Late Onset
Tardive dyskinesia*
Tardive dystonia
Rabbit syndrome

Idiosyncratic Effects
Urine may turn reddish with phenothiazines
Eye changes (pigmentary retinopathy); probably dose related
Agranulocytosis, other blood dyscrasias
Cholestatic jaundice
Skin rash, photosensitivity
Fetal toxicity has been reported with some agents
Electrocardiographic changes (prolonged QT interval) with some
agents

---

*Further information is found later in this section.
See also: Levinson DF, Simpson GM: Antipsychotic drug side effects. Psychiatr Update 6:704–723, 1987.

ANTIPSYCHOTIC AGENTS OF CHOICE FOR VARIOUS CONDITIONS

Condition	Recommended drug
Psychiatric	
Agitation and psychosis	Chlorpromazine, loxapine, mesoridazine, thioridazine
Withdrawal and psychosis	Fluphenazine, haloperidol, molindone, trifluoperazine
Suicidal tendency	Avoid mesoridazine and thioridazine
Tendency for severe parkinsonism or acute dystonia	Chlorpromazine, mesoridazine, thioridazine
Tendency for akathisia	Chlorpromazine, loxapine, mesoridazine, thioridazine
Elderly, medical history unknown, dehydration	Fluphenazine, haloperidol, molindone, perphenazine, thiothixene, trifluoperazine
Ophthalmologic	
Accommodation difficulties, Sjögren's syndrome	Fluphenazine, haloperidol, loxapine, molindone, perphenazine, prochlorperazine, thiothixene, trifluoperazine
Allergies	Chlorpromazine, loxapine, mesoridazine, thioridazine
Pulmonary	
Chronic obstructive pulmonary disease	Fluphenazine, haloperidol, loxapine, molindone, perphenazine, prochlorperazine, thiothixene, trifluoperazine

Cardiovascular

Coronary artery disease	Fluphenazine, haloperidol, molindone, perphenazine, thiothixene, trifluoperazine
Hypertension treated with prazosin	Fluphenazine, molindone, perphenazine, thiothixene, trifluoperazine
Arrhythmia	Avoid mesoridazine and thioridazine

Gastrointestinal

Nausea and vomiting	Any neuroleptic except thioridazine
Diarrhea	Chlorpromazine, mesoridazine, thioridazine

Urologic

Urinary retention	Fluphenazine, haloperidol, loxapine, molindone, perphenazine, prochlorperazine, thiothixene, trifluoperazine

Endocrinologic

Galactorrhea, menstrual irregularity caused by use of neuroleptic, breast cancer	Switch to chlorpromazine, loxapine, mesoridazine, molindone, thioridazine

Neurologic

Parkinson's disease	Chlorpromazine, mesoridazine, thioridazine
Delirium	Fluphenazine, haloperidol, molindone, perphenazine, thiothixene, trifluoperazine
Dementia with behavioral disorganization	Fluphenazine, haloperidol, molindone, perphenazine, thiothixene, trifluoperazine

From Black JL, Richelson E, Richardson JW: Antipsychotic agents: a clinical update. Mayo Clin Proc 60:777–789, 1985. By permission of Mayo Foundation.

DRUG INTERACTIONS WITH NEUROLEPTICS

Drug interacting with neuroleptic	Clinical effect of interaction
Anticholinergics	1. Delayed onset of neuroleptic effect in acute oral dose 2. May alter neuroleptic blood levels *3. Increased anticholinergic effect 4. Possible increased risk of hyperthermia
Antacids Cholestyramine Activated charcoal Kaolin Pectin	1. Oral absorption delayed
Lithium	1. May reduce chlorpromazine plasma levels and clinical effect *2. May increase central nervous system (CNS) toxicity
Phenytoin	1. May increase phenytoin toxicity 2. Decreased plasma levels and effect of neuroleptics
Opiates	*1. Increased sedation *2. Analgesia augmented *3. Hypotension augmented *4. Respiratory depression augmented *5. Anticholinergic effects augmented by meperidine
Benzodiazepines	1. Increased CNS sedation 2. Decreased akathisia
Cyclic antidepressants	*1. Increased sedation *2. Increased hypotension *3. Increased anticholinergic effect 4. May increase clinical effect of neuroleptic 5. Possible increased risk of seizures
L-Dopa	*1. May exacerbate psychosis *2. Decreased antiparkinsonian effect of L-dopa
Amphetamines	*1. May exacerbate psychosis by counteracting effects of neuroleptics

Drug interacting with neuroleptic	Clinical effect of interaction
Coffee Tea	1. Precipitates chlorpromazine in stomach; may delay clinical effect 2. May counteract sedation
Barbiturates Nonbarbiturate hypnotics	*1. Increased sedation *2. Decreased clinical effect of neuroleptic
Insulin Oral antidiabetic drugs	1. Neuroleptics increase blood glucose and may alter required dose of diabetic medication
Iproniazid	*1. Hepatic toxicity and encephalopathy *2. Decreased neuroleptic effect
Reserpine Clonidine Guanethidine Bethanidine Debrisoquine	*1. Decreased antihypertensive effect
Ammonium chloride	1. Decreased clinical effect of neuroleptics
Phenylpropanolamine	1. Ventricular arrhythmias with thioridazine 2. May increase sedation
Propranolol	*1. Increased blood levels of neuroleptic 2. Increased neurotoxicity 3. Increased neuroleptic effect 4. Seizure and cardiopulmonary arrest (case report)
Dichloralphenazone Rifampin Dioxyline Griseofulvin Phenylbutazone Carbamazepine	1. May decrease effect of neuroleptic by increasing metabolism
Chloramphenicol Disulfiram MAO inhibitors Oral contraceptives Acetaminophen	1. May increase effect of neuroleptic by inhibiting metabolism
Epinephrine	*1. Hypotension augmented

DRUG INTERACTIONS WITH NEUROLEPTICS—
continued

Drug interacting with neuroleptic	Clinical effect of interaction
Coumarin Phenindione	1. Generally may increase bleeding 2. Haloperidol may decrease bleeding via enzyme induction
Methyldopa	1. Reversible dementia with haloperidol 2. Increased sexual desire with chlorpromazine
Hydralazine Minoxidil	1. Enhanced hypotensive effect
Succinylcholine	1. May prolong apnea with ECT
Enflurane Isoflurane Anesthetics	*1. Profound hypotension with phenothiazines
Indomethacin	1. May cause severe drowsiness with haloperidol
Bromocriptine	1. Effects of bromocriptine are antagonized

*Indicates the interaction has caused clinically significant morbidity or mortality.
From Glassman R, Salzman C: Interactions beween psychotropic and other drugs: an update. Hosp Community Psychiatry 38:236–242, 1987. By permission of the American Psychiatric Association.

PROMINENT FEATURES OF TARDIVE DYSKINESIAS

Lingual-facial hyperkinesias
Chewing movements
Smacking and licking of the lips
Sucking movements
Tongue movements within the oral cavity
Tongue protrusion
Myokymic movements (worm-like movement on the surface of the tongue)
Blinking
Grotesque grimaces and spastic facial distortions

Neck and trunk movements
Spasmodic torticollis
Retrocollis
Torsion movements of the trunk
Axial hyperkinesia (hip rocking)

Choreoathetoid movements of the extremities

From Shader RI, Jackson AH: Approaches to schizophrenia, in Manual of Psychiatric Therapeutics: Practical Psychopharmacology and Psychiatry. Edited by Shader RI. Boston, MA, Little, Brown, 1975, pp 63–100. By permission of the publisher.

ABNORMAL INVOLUNTARY MOVEMENT SCALE (AIMS)

Examination Procedure

Either before or after completing the examination procedure, unobtrusively observe the patient at rest (e.g., in waiting room).

The chair to be used in this examination should be firm and without arms.

For each observation, the patient is rated on a scale of 0 (none), 1 (minimal), 2 (mild), 3 (moderate), or 4 (severe) according to the severity of symptoms.

1. Ask the patient whether there is anything in his/her mouth (i.e., gum, candy, etc.) and if there is, to remove it.

2. Ask patient about the *current* condition of his/her teeth. Ask patient if he/she wears dentures. Do teeth or dentures bother patient *now*?
3. Ask patient whether he/she notices any movements in mouth, face, hands, or feet. If yes, ask to describe and to what extent they *currently* bother patient or interfere with his/her activities.
4. Ask patient to remove his/her shoes. Have patient sit in chair with hands on knees, legs slightly apart, and feet flat on floor. (Look at entire body for movements in this position.)
5. Ask patient to sit with hands hanging unsupported. If male, between legs, if female and wearing a dress, hanging over knees. (Observe hands and other body areas.)
6. Ask patient to open mouth. (Observe tongue at rest within mouth.) Do this twice.
7. Ask patient to protrude tongue. (Observe abnormalities of tongue movement.) Do this twice.
8. Ask the patient to tap thumb, with each finger, as rapidly as possible for 10–15 seconds—separately with right hand, then with left hand. (Observe facial and leg movements.)*
9. Flex and extend patient's left and right arms (one at a time).
10. Ask patient to stand up. (Observe in profile. Observe all body areas again, hips included.)
11. Ask patient to extend both arms in front with palms down. (Observe trunk, legs, and mouth.)*
12. Have patient walk a few paces, turn, and walk back to chair. (Observe hands and gait.) Do this twice.*

---

*Activated movements.

From Guy W: ECDEU Assessment Manual for Psychopharmacology, Revised, 1976. U.S. Department of Health, Education, and Welfare, Public Health Service, 1976, p 535.

Rating Procedure for the Abnormal Involuntary Movement Scale (AIMS)

MOVEMENT RATINGS: Rate highest severity observed. Rate movements that occur upon activation one point *less* than those observed spontaneously.

Code:
0 = None
1 = Minimal, may be extreme normal
2 = Mild
3 = Moderate
4 = Severe

Score 0–4

FACIAL AND ORAL MOVEMENTS:

1. Muscles of Facial Expression
   e.g., movements of forehead, eyebrows, periorbital area, cheeks; include frowning, blinking, smiling, grimacing

2. Lips and Perioral Area
   e.g., puckering, pouting, smacking

3. Jaw
   e.g., biting, clenching, chewing, mouth opening, lateral movement

4. Tongue
   Rate only increase in movement both in and out of mouth, NOT inability to sustain movement

EXTREMITY MOVEMENTS:

5. Upper (arms, wrists, hands, fingers)
   Include choreic movements (i.e., rapid, objectively purposeless, irregular, spontaneous), athetoid movements (i.e., slow, irregular, complex, serpentine)
   Do NOT include tremor (i.e., repetitive, regular, rhythmic)

6. Lower (legs, knees, ankles, toes)
   e.g., lateral knee movement, foot tapping, heel dropping, foot squirming, inversion and eversion of foot

TRUNK MOVEMENTS:

7. Neck, shoulders, hips
   e.g., rocking, twisting, squirming, pelvic gyrations

8. Severity of abnormal movements

GLOBAL JUDGMENTS:

9. Incapacitation due to abnormal movements

10. Patient's awareness of abnormal movements
    Rate only patient's report

DENTAL STATUS:	11. Current problems with teeth and/or dentures	No	0
		Yes	1
	12. Does patient usually wear dentures?	No	0
		Yes	1

From Guy W: ECDEU Assessment Manual for Psychopharmacology, Revised, 1976. U.S. Department of Health, Education, and Welfare, Public Health Service, 1976, p 534.

NEUROLEPTIC MALIGNANT SYNDROME

Signs and Symptoms
Hyperthermia
Muscle rigidity
Mental status changes
Dysautonomia: pallor/flushing
                 instability of blood pressure
                 diaphoresis
                 tachycardia
Infrequent: trismus
            opisthotonos
            seizures
            . Babinski sign

Laboratory Findings
Elevated serum creatine phosphokinase (CPK)
Leukocytosis
Elevated serum liver function tests
May see: Rhabdomyolysis and myoglobinuria
May see: Dehydration and electrolyte changes

Differential Diagnosis
Heat stroke
Catatonia
Monoamine oxidase inhibitor (MAOI) crisis
Malignant hyperthermia with anesthesia
Central anticholinergic syndrome

Management

1. Monitor vital signs and mental status closely
2. Stop neuroleptics
3. Intravenous hydration; cooling blankets for hyperthermia
4. Rule out possible infection (blood, urine, cerebrospinal fluid)
5. Monitor serum CPK every 12 hours
6. Monitor fluids and electrolytes
7. Transfer to intensive care unit if necessary
8. Pharmacotherapy may include use of: Dantrolene
   Bromocriptine
   Pancuronium bromide
   Amantadine
   Nifedipine

Modified from Guzé BH, Baxter LR Jr: Current concepts: neuroleptic malignant syndrome. N Engl J Med 313:163–166, 1985.
See also: Levenson JL: Neuroleptic malignant syndrome. Am J Psychiatry 142:1137–1145, 1985.

ANTIPARKINSONIAN DRUGS FOR TREATMENT OF EXTRAPYRAMIDAL SYMPTOMS

Generic name	Trade name	Typical dosage
Tropine derivatives		
benztropine	Cogentin	1–4 mg q12–24h
Piperidine compounds		
biperiden	Akineton	2 mg q8–24h
procyclidine	Kemadrin	2.5 mg q8h
trihexyphenidyl	Artane	5 mg q8–24h
Ethanolamine antihistamines		
diphenhydramine	Benadryl	25–50 mg q6–8h
orphenadrine	Norflex	100 mg q12h
Antiviral agent		
amantadine	Symmetrel	100 mg q12–24h

Modified from Shader RI, Jackson AH: Approaches to schizophrenia, in Manual of Psychiatric Therapeutics: Practical Psychopharmacology and Psychiatry. Edited by Shader RI. Boston, MA, Little, Brown, 1975, pp 63–100.

SIDE EFFECTS OF ANTIPARKINSONIAN AGENTS

Generally, these agents are antihistaminic and antimuscarinic. Prominent side effects include dry mouth, urinary hesitancy, blurred vision, constipation, decreased sweating, mydriasis, exacerbation or onset of narrow-angle glaucoma, sedation, and memory dysfunction. Ileus can be a late sign of anticholinergic toxicity.

Amantadine, also used as an antiviral agent, may cause livedo reticularis, restlessness, confusion, hallucinations, and, rarely, convulsions. It does not have antihistaminic or antimuscarinic effects.

Central anticholinergic toxicity syndrome is characterized by confusion, anxiety, restlessness, hallucinations, or delirium. Other clinical signs include fever, flushing, dilated pupils, constipation, and decreased secretions. Seizures or coma may follow. (A useful mnemonic is, "mad as a hatter, red as a beet, and dry as a bone.") Sudden change in mental status following the initiation of anticholinergic therapy should be assessed. Physostigmine can reverse these effects if treatment for severe toxicity is required. Patients must be closely monitored because physostigmine may induce seizures.

ANTIDEPRESSANT DRUGS

CLINICAL GUIDELINES FOR USE OF ANTIDEPRESSANTS

1. Appropriate choice: select on the basis of the profile of side effects, particularly sedative effects in agitated patients, or on the basis of previous response or family history of response to a particular agent.
2. Adequate dose: check blood level if toxicity ensues or after 3 weeks if response is inadequate.
3. Adequate duration: administer for a minimum of 4 months after recovery.
4. Adequate termination or maintenance: for first depression, 4–5 months after recovery, taper dose gradually for 4–8 weeks and then discontinue therapy. For recurrent unipolar depression, maintain antidepressant therapy. Optimal maintenance dose is usually at least half of the initial therapeutic dose.
5. Adequate therapy: for almost all types of depression, a combina-

tion of psychotherapy and antidepressants may be more effective than antidepressants alone.

6. Alternatives: change antidepressant class; add lithium; add synthetic thyroid; add stimulant; combine tricyclic and monoamine oxidase inhibitor (avoid imipramine); intensify psychotherapy; or use electroshock therapy (the most effective treatment).

Modified from Richardson JW III, Richelson E: Antidepressants: a clinical update for medical practitioners. Mayo Clin Proc 59:330–337, 1984.

DAILY DOSES AND PROJECTED THERAPEUTIC PLASMA RANGES OF TRICYCLIC AND OTHER ANTIDEPRESSANTS

For any of the listed antidepressants, elderly persons should be treated with about half of the recommended dosage for adults. Dosage should be divided initially. If side effects are tolerated, all heterocyclic antidepressants may be prescribed as one daily dose. (Fluoxetine and bupropion are not heterocyclic antidepressants and are exceptions.)

Drug (generic and trade names)	Usual daily dose for adults (mg)	Dosage range (mg/day)	Projected optimal therapeutic plasma range (ng/ml)
Tricyclic: tertiary amines			
Amitriptyline (Elavil, Endep)	150–200	50–300	80–250*
Doxepin (Adapin, Sinequan)	75–150	50–300	150–250*
Imipramine (Tofranil)	75–150	50–300	150–250*
Trimipramine (Surmontil)	100–200	50–300	150–250
Tricyclic: secondary amines			
Desipramine (Norpramin, Pertofrane)	100–200	50–300	125–300
Nortriptyline (Pamelor)	50–100	30–125	50–150
Protriptyline (Vivactil)	15–40	10–60	70–260
Dibenzoxazepine			
Amoxapine (Asendin)	200–300	50–400	200–600*

DAILY DOSES AND PROJECTED THERAPEUTIC PLASMA RANGES OF TRICYCLIC AND OTHER ANTIDEPRESSANTS— continued

Drug (generic and trade names)	Usual daily dose for adults (mg)	Dosage range (mg/day)	Projected optimal therapeutic plasma range (ng/ml)
Tetracyclic			
Maprotiline (Ludiomil)	100–150	50–225	200–600
Triazolopyridine			
Trazodone (Desyrel)	150–400	50–600	800–1,600
Benzene propanamine			
Fluoxetine (Prozac)	20–60	20–80	...
Aminoketone			
Bupropion (Wellbutrin)	300	200–450	...

*Level is for administered drug and active metabolite (i.e., amitriptyline + nortriptyline, doxepin + desmethyldoxepin, imipramine + desipramine, amoxapine + 7-hydroxyamoxapine + 8-hydroxyamoxapine).

Modified from Richelson E: Antidepressants: pharmacology and clinical use, in Treatments of Psychiatric Disorders. Edited by Karasu TB. Washington, DC, American Psychiatric Association, 1989, pp 1773–1787. By permission of the publisher.

SIDE EFFECTS OF HETEROCYCLIC ANTIDEPRESSANTS

Antimuscarinic effects
Dry mouth
Constipation
Urinary hesitancy
Blurred vision (loss of accommodation)
Confusion, memory disturbance
Sinus tachycardia
Exacerbation of narrow-angle glaucoma

Antihistaminic effects
Drowsiness
Weight gain

Anti-α-adrenergic effects
Orthostatic hypotension

Other
Galactorrhea, extrapyramidal symptoms (especially with amoxapine)
Quinidine-like cardiac conduction changes
Skin rash, photosensitivity with some agents
Seizures
Precipitation of mania
Priapism (especially with trazodone)
Rare: Agranulocytosis, thrombocytopenia
Liver necrosis

See also:

Blackwell B: Side effects of antidepressant drugs. Psychiatr Update 6:724–745, 1987.
Baldessarini RJ: Current status of antidepressants: clinical pharmacology and therapy. J Clin Psychiatry 50:117–126, 1989.

PREFERRED ANTIDEPRESSANTS WHEN SPECIFIC MEDICAL DISORDERS COEXIST WITH DEPRESSION

I. **Cardiovascular**
   A. Congestive heart failure or coronary artery disease—nortriptyline
   B. Conduction defect—maprotiline
   C. Hypertension treated with guanethidine or guanadrel—trazodone, trimipramine, fluoxetine
   D. Hypertension treated with prazosin—fluoxetine, desipramine, protriptyline
   E. Hypertension treated with clonidine, guanabenz, or α-methyldopa—fluoxetine, maprotiline
   F. Untreated mild hypertension—imipramine, monoamine oxidase inhibitor
   G. Postural hypotension—maprotiline, fluoxetine, nortriptyline (avoid imipramine and amitriptyline)

II.   **Neurologic**
   A. Seizure disorder—monoamine oxidase inhibitor best; secondary amine (e.g., desipramine) better than tertiary amine (e.g., imipramine); avoid maprotiline, amoxapine, trimipramine, bupropion
   B. Organic brain syndrome—trazodone, fluoxetine, amoxapine, maprotiline, desipramine
   C. Chronic pain syndrome—amitriptyline, doxepin
   D. Migraine headaches—trazodone, doxepin, trimipramine, amitriptyline
   E. Psychosis—antidepressant plus neuroleptic, amoxapine
   F. Parkinsonism—amitriptyline, protriptyline, trimipramine, doxepin, imipramine; avoid amoxapine
   G. Tardive dyskinesia—trazodone, desipramine, doxepin, imipramine; avoid amoxapine

III. **Allergic**—doxepin, amitriptyline, trimipramine, imipramine, nortriptyline

IV.   **Gastrointestinal**
   A. Chronic diarrhea—doxepin, trimipramine, amitriptyline, imipramine, protriptyline
   B. Chronic constipation—trazodone, fluoxetine, amoxapine, maprotiline, desipramine
   C. Peptic ulcer disease—doxepin, trimipramine, amitriptyline, imipramine

V.   **Urologic**
   A. Neurogenic bladder—trazodone, fluoxetine, amoxapine, maprotiline, desipramine
   B. Organic impotence—trazodone, fluoxetine, amoxapine, maprotiline, desipramine

VI.   **Ophthalmologic** (angle-closure glaucoma)—trazodone, fluoxetine, amoxapine, maprotiline, desipramine

---

Modified from Richardson JW III, Richelson E: Antidepressants: a clinical update for medical practitioners. Mayo Clin Proc 59:330–337, 1984.

DRUG INTERACTIONS WITH CYCLIC ANTIDEPRESSANTS

Drug interacting with antidepressant	Clinical effect of interaction
Cimetidine Methylphenidate Acetaminophen Oral contraceptives Chloramphenicol Isoniazid MAO inhibitors	*1. Inhibits metabolism, increasing blood levels and toxicity of antidepressants
Disulfiram	1. Inhibits metabolism, increasing blood levels of antidepressants 2. Possible induction of psychosis and confusional state
Guanethidine Debrisoquine Bethanidine	*1. Decreased antihypertensive effect 2. Decreased antidepressant effect
Clonidine	1. Decreased antihypertensive and antidepressant effect 2. Potential hypertensive crisis with imipramine (case report)
Thiazide diuretics Acetazolamide	1. Hypotension augmented
Quinidine Procainamide	*1. Cardiac conduction prolonged
Methyldopa	1. Increased agitation, tremor, tachycardia
Propranolol	1. Decreased antidepressant effect
Coumarin anticoagulants	*1. Increased bleeding
Neuroleptics	1. Antidepressants may increase plasma level of neuroleptic
Anticholinergic drugs	1. Increased anticholinergic toxicity

DRUG INTERACTIONS
WITH CYCLIC ANTIDEPRESSANTS—continued

Drug interacting with antidepressant	Clinical effect of interaction
Phenytoin Barbiturates Nonbarbiturate hypnotics Dichloralphenazone Rifampin Doxycycline Griseofulvin Carbamazepine Phenylbutazone	*1. Induces hepatic metabolism, decreasing clinical effect of antidepressants
Triiodothyronine (T_3) Lithium	1. Possible potentiation of antidepressant effect
Activated charcoal Kaolin	1. Helpful in overdose by decreasing absorption
Estrogen	1. Decreased therapeutic effect of imipramine 2. Lethargy, headache, hypotension 3. Akathisia
Testosterone	1. Paranoid psychosis with aggression
Halothane Enflurane Anesthetics	1. Tachycardia with imipramine
Phenytoin Phenylbutazone Aspirin Aminopyrine Scopolamine	1. Increased antidepressant effect by displacement from protein binding sites
Epinephrine Local anesthetic dissolved in epinephrine	*1. Hypotension augmented *2. Increased bleeding in nasal surgery
Benzodiazepines	*1. Increased CNS sedation, increased confusion, decreased motor functions 2. Increased suicide risk

Drug interacting with antidepressant	Clinical effect of interaction
Phenothiazines	1. Increased tricyclic levels 2. Possible ventricular arrhythmias with thioridazine with combination of drugs
L-Dopa	1. Increased agitation, tremor, rigidity are possible 2. Decreased plasma levels of antidepressants via impaired gastrointestinal absorption
Alcohol	1. Increased sedation

*Indicates interaction that has caused clinically significant morbidity or mortality.
From Glassman R, Salzman C: Interactions between psychotropic and other drugs: an update. Hosp Community Psychiatry 38:236–242, 1987. By permission of the American Psychiatric Association.

MONOAMINE OXIDASE INHIBITORS

Drug	Trade name	Usual therapeutic dose range (mg/day)
Isocarboxazid	Marplan	10–30
Phenelzine	Nardil	30–90
Tranylcypromine	Parnate	30–60

Modified from Schatzberg AF, Cole JO: Manual of Clinical Psychopharmacology. Washington, DC, American Psychiatric Press, 1986, p 48.

SIDE EFFECTS OF MONOAMINE OXIDASE INHIBITORS (MAOIs)

Atropine-like Effects

Dry mouth   Urinary hesitancy
Blurred vision   Constipation
Drowsiness

Cardiovascular

Lightheadedness   Peripheral edema
Orthostatic hypotension

Other Side Effects

Restlessness/insomnia/anorexia   Flushing/sweating
Nightmares   Skin rash/purpura
Decreased sexual potency   Hallucinations/hypomania
Ejaculatory disturbances   Myoclonic twitches
Tiredness/weakness

Acute Toxicity Reaction (Hypertensive Crisis)

Nausea and vomiting
Sweating
Severe occipital headache/pounding headache
Stiff neck/sore neck
Palpitations/tachycardia/bradycardia
Chest pain
Seizure

Management: Discontinue MAOI and reduce blood pressure—phentolamine, 5–10 mg iv, may be given slowly. For mild cases, observation and blood pressure monitoring may suffice. Sublingual nifedipine has also been used (Clary C, Schweizer E: Treatment of MAOI hypertensive crisis with sublingual nifedipine. J Clin Psychiatry 48:249–250, 1987).

See also: Blackwell B: Side effects of antidepressant drugs. Psychiatr Update 6:724–745, 1987.

DRUG INTERACTIONS WITH MONOAMINE OXIDASE INHIBITORS (MAOIs)

Drug interacting with MAOIs	Clinical effect of interaction
Amphetamines Ephedrine Metaraminol Levarterenol Methylphenidate Phenylephrine Pseudoephedrine L-Dopa Dopamine Mephentermine Chlorpheniramine Procaine (dissolved in epinephrine)	*1. Increased blood pressure
Cyclic antidepressants	1. May have enhanced clinical effect *2. Conflicting reports on toxicity—hyperpyrexia, hypertension, excitability, muscle rigidity, convulsions, coma; use with caution 3. Weight gain
Meperidine	*1. Excitation, sweating, hypotension; use other narcotics; can be life threatening
Succinylcholine	1. Phenelzine may prolong apnea with electroconvulsive therapy
General anesthetics Anticholinergics Sedative-hypnotics Antihistamines Benzodiazepines	1. May enhance central nervous system (CNS) depression
Insulin Sulfonylurea Phenformin	1. Increased hypotension
Thiazide diuretics Hydralazine Phenothiazines Reserpine	1. Increased hypotension
Guanethidine	1. Decreased antihypertensive effect

DRUG INTERACTIONS WITH MONOAMINE OXIDASE INHIBITORS (MAOIs)—continued

Drug interacting with MAOIs	Clinical effect of interaction
Methyldopa	1. Excitation, visual hallucinations with pargyline
Alcohol	1. Decreased MAO inhibition
	2. CNS depression

*Indicates interaction that has caused clinically significant morbidity or mortality.
From Glassman R, Salzman C: Interactions between psychotropic and other drugs: an update. Hosp Community Psychiatry 38:236–242, 1987. By permission of the American Psychiatric Association.

FOOD RESTRICTIONS FOR PATIENTS TAKING MONOAMINE OXIDASE INHIBITORS (MAOIs)

Food containing large amounts of tyramine or dopamine may cause a hypertensive crisis if ingested by patients taking MAOIs. Patients should be cautioned about foods rich in these amines and about foods prepared by means of protein breakdown (such as smoking, pickling, fermenting, aging, or treating with bacteria), which may release biologically active amines. Spoiled, unfresh, and contaminated foods must be avoided.

Coffee, tea, and cola-type beverages do not contain tyramine but have some stimulant activity which may cause a pressor effect. These beverages should be consumed in moderation. Chocolate is permissible except in excessive quantities.

Alcoholic beverages (other than beer, liqueurs, red wines, vermouth, and sherries, which should be avoided) may be consumed, but only in moderation, because they may cause excessive sedation when combined with MAOIs.

It is important to warn patients about the pharmacologic interaction of MAOIs with over-the-counter, illicit, and prescription drugs. These highly potent agents are more likely to cause dangerous interactions than most foods. Harrison et al. noted that over-the-counter remedies may have both safe and unsafe formulations with similar names (Harrison WM, McGrath PJ, Stewart JW, et al: MAOIs and hypertensive crises: the role of OTC drugs. J Clin Psychol 50:64–65, 1989).

Hierarchical Ordering of Restricted Foods for a Low-Tyramine Diet

Restricted items	Comment
Foodstuffs to avoid	
Cheese	Cottage, processed American, and cream cheese permitted
Beer, red wine, sherry, and liqueurs	Clear spirits and white wine permitted
Yeast/protein extracts	
Includes some packet soups and yeast vitamin supplements (brewers' yeast)	
Fava or broad bean pods (Italian green beans)	Shelled beans or other legumes permitted
Smoked or pickled fish (herring, caviar)	
Beef or chicken liver	
Fermented sausage (bologna, pepperoni, salami, summer sausage)	
Canned or overripe figs	
Stewed whole bananas (banana peel)	Banana pulp permitted
Sauerkraut	
Foodstuffs to consider; less likely to pose problems	
Other meats	Meats should be fresh
Other alcoholic beverages	Consume in moderation
Yogurt and sour cream	Consume reputable brand in moderation
Avocado/guacamole	Consume in moderation
New Zealand spinach	Consume in moderation
Soy sauce	Consume in moderation
Fruits	Avoid overripe fruit

Modified from Folks DG: Monoamine oxidase inhibitors: reappraisal of dietary considerations. J Clin Psychopharmacol 3:249–252, 1983.
See also: Foods interacting with MAO inhibitors. Med Lett Drugs Ther 31:11–12, 1989.

LITHIUM

SIDE EFFECTS OF LITHIUM

Early Onset and Often Transient
Gastrointestinal upset (nausea, cramps, diarrhea)

Hand tremor   Thirst

Muscle weakness   Headache

Fatigue/insomnia   Decreased concentration

Variable Onset
Cogwheeling

Hypothyroidism/increased thyroid-stimulating hormone (TSH)

Weight gain

Polyuria/polydipsia

Pseudohyperparathyroidism

Leukocytosis

T-wave suppression (lithium is contraindicated in sick sinus syndrome)

Skin rashes

Therapeutic Level
Initial: 0.8–1.3 mEq/L (maintenance 0.5–0.8 mEq/L)

Toxicity
At blood levels >1.5 mEq/L (in some patients, may occur at therapeutic plasma levels)

With increasing toxicity see progression of

Fatigue/lassitude $\longrightarrow$ Mental blunting $\longrightarrow$ Ataxia $\longrightarrow$ Stupor $\longrightarrow$ Coma

Tremor $\longrightarrow$ Jerking $\longrightarrow$ Increased deep tendon reflexes $\longrightarrow$ Seizure

Levels > 4.0 mEq/L are potentially fatal

Teratogenic (cardiac anomalies)

See also:

Jefferson JW, Greist JH: Lithium carbonate and carbamazepine side effects. Psychiatr Update 6:746–780, 1987.

Jefferson JW, Greist JH, Ackerman DL, et al: Lithium Encyclopedia for Clinical Practice, 2nd Edition. Washington, DC, American Psychiatric Press, 1987.

Schou M: Lithium prophylaxis: myths and realities. Am J Psychol 146:573–576, 1989.

DRUG INTERACTIONS WITH LITHIUM

Drug interacting with lithium	Clinical effect of interaction
Indomethacin Piroxicam Sulindac Ibuprofen Phenylbutazone Naproxen	*1. Increased lithium effect and toxicity due to decreased renal lithium clearance
Thiazide diuretics Spironolactone Triamterene Amiloride	*1. Increased lithium effect and toxicity due to decreased renal lithium clearance
Neuroleptics	1. Decreased neuroleptic blood levels 2. Decreased nausea and vomiting from lithium 3. Increased neurotoxicity (may be severe)†
Phenytoin	1. May increase neurotoxicity of both drugs
Theophylline Acetazolamide Aminophylline	*1. Increased renal excretion of lithium, decreasing its effect
Succinylcholine Pancuronium Decamethonium	1. Prolonged apnea with electroconvulsive therapy (ECT)†
Amphetamines	1. May increase amphetamine "high"
Benzodiazepines	1. Hypothermia associated with diazepam (case report)
Potassium iodide	1. Increased likelihood of hypothyroidism
Sodium bicarbonate Sodium chloride Urea Mannitol	*1. Increased renal excretion of lithium, decreasing its effect

DRUG INTERACTIONS WITH LITHIUM—continued

Drug interacting with lithium	Clinical effect of interaction
Tetracycline Spectinomycin	*1. Increased lithium effect and toxicity due to decreased renal lithium clearance
Carbamazepine	1. Increased neurotoxicity of both drugs 2. Increased polyuria, ataxia, and dizziness due to antidiuretic property of carbamazepine
Cyclic antidepressants	1. May increase lithium neurotoxicity 2. May increase lithium tremor
Ketamine	*1. Increased lithium toxicity resulting from sodium depletion
Digitalis	1. May cause cardiac arrhythmia by depleting intracellular potassium
Furosemide	*1. Increased lithium toxicity resulting from sodium depletion
Insulin	1. Insulin dosage may need adjustment early in lithium treatment due to altered glucose tolerance
Mazindol	1. Increased lithium toxicity
Norepinephrine	1. Decreased pressor response to norepinephrine

*Indicates interaction that has caused clinically significant morbidity or mortality.
†Some physicians dispute the clinical significance of this effect.
From Glassman R, Salzman C: Interactions between psychotropic and other drugs: an update. Hosp Community Psychiatry 38:236–242, 1987. By permission of the American Psychiatric Association.

CARBAMAZEPINE

SIDE EFFECTS OF CARBAMAZEPINE

Dermatologic
Itching, hives, rashes, sores in mouth, mild eczema, exfoliative dermatitis, Stevens-Johnson syndrome, aggravation of systemic lupus erythematosus (SLE)

Hematologic
Commonly see leukopenia to 3,000–5,000 leukocytes/μl; rarely see thrombocytopenia or anemia; eosinophilia, agranulocytosis, and aplastic anemia have been reported; fatalities have occurred; stop drug therapy if the combination of eosinophilia with rash, chills/fever, arthralgia/myalgia, and lymphadenopathy occurs; check complete blood count when initiating treatment; monitor regularly

Hepatic
Chemical hepatitis, cholestatic jaundice

Cardiovascular
Hypotension, hypertension, congestive heart failure, syncope, edema, thrombophlebitis

Genitourinary
Urinary retention, frequency, impotence

Central Nervous System
Dizziness, fatigue, incoordination, visual disturbance, speech disturbance, tinnitus, depression

Other
Gastrointestinal distress, arthralgia, lymphadenopathy

Therapeutic Level (for anticonvulsant activity): 4–12 μg/ml. Therapeutic level for mood-stabilizing effect is not known; some authors suggest it is less than that required for anticonvulsant activity.

See also: Jefferson JW, Greist JH: Lithium carbonate and carbamazepine side effects. Psychiatr Update 6:746–780, 1987.

DRUG INTERACTIONS WITH CARBAMAZEPINE

Drug interacting with carbamazepine	Clinical effect of interaction
Lithium	1. Inhibits diuresis and polyuria associated with lithium *2. In combination, may increase ataxia, feelings of unreality, dizziness *3. Neurotoxicity with normal levels of both
Haloperidol	1. May decrease carbamazepine levels and vice versa
Cimetidine Erythromycin Isoniazid	1. Increased carbamazepine levels *2. May produce somnolence, lethargy, nystagmus, dizziness, nausea, vomiting in combination
Propoxyphene	*1. Increased carbamazepine levels 2. May produce headache, dizziness, nausea, ataxia
Clonazepam	1. Clonazepam levels decreased by carbamazepine
Charcoal	1. Binds carbamazepine; good for use in overdose
Phenytoin	1. Decreased carbamazepine levels, but carbamazepine does not affect phenytoin levels
Phenobarbital Primidone	1. Decreased carbamazepine levels
Corticosteroids Coumarin anticoagulants Doxycycline Oral contraceptives	1. Decreased effect of carbamazepine
Verapamil	1. Increased carbamazepine toxicity, especially neurotoxicity

*Indicates interaction that has caused clinically significant morbidity or mortality.
From Glassman R, Salzman C: Interactions between psychotropic and other drugs: an update. Hosp Community Psychiatry 38:236–242, 1987. By permission of the American Psychiatric Association.

BENZODIAZEPINES

POTENCY AND PHARMACOKINETICS OF BENZODIAZEPINES

Generic name	Trade name	Average daily oral dose range (mg)	Approx. dose needed to achieve anxiolytic effect of 5 mg diazepam (mg)*	Half-life (h)
Alprazolam	Xanax	0.75–4	0.5	6–20
Chlordiaze-poxide	Librium	15–40	10	5–30†
Clonazepam	Klonopin	0.25–1.5	0.25	18–50
Clorazepate	Tranxene	15–30	7.5	†
Diazepam	Valium	5–30	5	20–100†
Flurazepam	Dalmane	15–30	15	†
Halazepam	Paxipam	80–160	20	14†
Lorazepam	Ativan	1–6	1	10–20
Midazolam	Versed	1–5	1	1–12
Oxazepam	Serax	45–120	15	4–15
Prazepam	Centrax	20–60	10	†
Temazepam	Restoril	10–40	15	8–22
Triazolam	Halcion	0.25–0.5	0.25	2–3

*Clinical equivalence for anxiolysis and sedation may differ.
†Active metabolites may extend half-life to 60 hours or more.

SIDE EFFECTS OF BENZODIAZEPINES

These are sedative agents and generally interact in a synergistic way with other central nervous system depressants (e.g., alcohol and barbiturates). Benzodiazepines are metabolized in the liver; this may be slowed in the elderly or in persons with liver disease. These agents are addictive. Insomnia, rebound anxiety, recurrence of original anxiety symptoms, and other withdrawal symptoms may complicate discontinuing benzodiazepine therapy.

Central Nervous System
Drowsiness, lightheadedness, ataxia, fatigue, weakness
More rarely: confusion, hallucinations, depression, amnesia
Paradoxical stimulation has occurred and is characterized by anxiety, tremor, insomnia, rage, hyperactivity (especially in children)

Other (infrequent)
GI complaints (constipation, diarrhea, cramps, nausea)
Dry mouth
Urinary hesitancy
Skin changes (rash, pruritus, photosensitivity, hypersensitivity reactions)
Visual disturbances

See also: Rickels K, Schweizer E, Lucki I: Benzodiazepine side effects. Psychiatr Update 6:781–801, 1987.

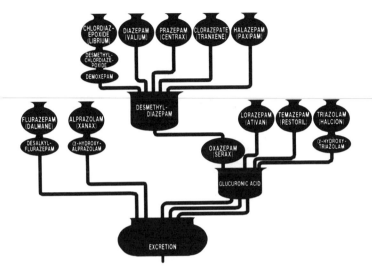

Major routes of metabolism of benzodiazepines

DRUG INTERACTIONS WITH BENZODIAZEPINES

Drug interacting with benzodiazepine	Clinical effect of interaction
Cimetidine Isoniazid Disulfiram Oral contraceptives	1. Increased toxicity of diazepam and chlordiazepoxide due to inhibition of metabolism
Rifampin Phenytoin	1. Decreased clinical effect due to induced hepatic metabolism 2. Increased level of phenytoin
Antacids Anticholinergics	1. Delay in oral absorption
Digoxin	1. Increased digoxin levels
Alcohol Neuroleptics Narcotics Antihistamines Sedative-hypnotics	*1. Increased central nervous system (CNS) sedation 2. Increased level of diazepam and chlordiazepoxide with alcohol
Cyclic antidepressants	1. Increased CNS sedation 2. Increased amitriptyline, imipramine, desipramine levels
L-Dopa	1. Possible decreased effect of L-dopa
Erythromycin	1. Increased level of triazolam

*Indicates interaction that has caused clinically significant morbidity or mortality.
Modified from Glassman R, Salzman C: Interactions between psychotropic and other drugs: an update. Hosp Community Psychiatry 38:236–242, 1987.

CENTRAL NERVOUS SYSTEM STIMULANTS

SIDE EFFECTS OF CENTRAL NERVOUS SYSTEM (CNS) STIMULANTS

This class of agents includes the amphetamines and other CNS stimulants such as methylphenidate and pemoline. They are useful in the treatment of attention-deficit hyperactivity disorder and narcolepsy and as adjunctive treatment in some depressive disorders. Several CNS stimulants are potential drugs of abuse: cocaine is an example. Potency varies greatly among individuals due to variation in absorption, metabolism, and tolerance.

Principal side effects include irritability, restlessness, motor agitation, insomnia, anorexia, and tremor. Some patients, especially children, may report nausea and abdominal pain. Paranoia may occur with large doses.

Other Effects
Exacerbation of motor tics (unmasking of Tourette's syndrome)
Increased blood pressure, tachycardia
Cardiac arrhythmias at larger doses
Dry mouth
Growth suppression with long-term use in children; growth is restored when drug therapy is stopped
Rare: suppression of leukocytes, altered hepatic function
Withdrawal of medication is notable for depressed mood and lethargy; this depression often responds to tricyclic antidepressants

β-ADRENERGIC BLOCKERS

SIDE EFFECTS OF β-ADRENERGIC BLOCKERS

The β-adrenergic blockers (e.g., propranolol, metoprolol) are useful in the treatment of anxiety disorders and for organic personality disorder (explosive type). Principal side effects include bradycardia, hypotension, bronchospasm, intensification of atrioventricular block, and depression; rarely, vivid dreams and hallucinations occur. The dosage of β-blockers should always be tapered when the drug is discontinued in order to avoid rebound hypertension.

Contraindications include asthma, Raynaud's syndrome, sinus bradycardia and other arrhythmias, congestive heart failure, and malignant hypertension. β-Blockers should be used with caution in the presence of diabetes mellitus or thyroid dysfunction.

Drug interactions include synergistic effects with other antihypertensive agents, although use with methyldopa leads to hypertension through unopposed α-adrenergic stimulation. β-Blockers cause increased plasma levels of antipsychotics, hypotension with monoamine oxidase inhibitors, and additive effects with some antiarrhythmic agents (e.g., verapamil).

See also:

Jenkins SC, Maruta T: Therapeutic use of propranolol for intermittent explosive disorder. Mayo Clin Proc 62:204–214, 1987.

Lader M: β-Adrenoceptor antagonists in neuropsychiatry: an update. J Clin Psychiatry 49:213–223, 1988.

Yudofsky SC, Silver JM: Psychiatric aspects of brain injury: trauma, stroke and tumor. Psychiatr Update 4:142–158, 1985.

DISULFIRAM

SIDE EFFECTS OF DISULFIRAM

Generally Transient
Fatigue, headache, allergic dermatitis, metallic taste, drowsiness

Variable Onset
Vertigo, insomnia, personality change, dysarthria, seizure, peripheral neuropathy, halitosis, impotence, confusion/psychosis/seizure, hypersensitivity, hepatitis, fetal malformation, blood dyscrasias

Drug Interactions
Disulfiram inhibits hepatic metabolism and increases the clinical effect or toxicity of many agents. The most important interactions are with warfarin, phenytoin, isoniazid, metronidazole, and perphenazine. Concurrent use of these agents should be avoided.

Disulfiram elevates blood levels of benzodiazepines, with the exception of oxazepam.

Disulfiram/Alcohol Reaction

Many liquid nonprescription and prescription remedies contain alcohol as a vehicle and should be avoided. This should also be considered with some personal hygiene products and cosmetics.

Alcohol toxicity reaction consists of flushing, sweating, palpitations, tachycardia, hyperventilation, throbbing headache, hypotension, vertigo, blurred vision, weakness, nausea/vomiting, and electrocardiographic changes. It is generally self-limited; however, severe reactions have resulted in death. If the reaction is severe, monitor electrocardiogram, respiration, blood pressure, and electrolytes, and treat as for shock.

CHEMICAL DEPENDENCE

This section is organized by major categories of drugs of abuse: cannabis, central nervous system (CNS) depressants and alcohol, CNS stimulants, hallucinogens, opiates, volatile inhalants, and anticholinergics. Each category includes:

Agents
Street Names (highly variable with time and region of use)
Intoxication Syndromes
Management of Intoxication
Withdrawal Syndromes
Management of Withdrawal
Medical Complications of Chronic Use

These sections are expanded, and extra tables are included where necessary to convey appropriate information (e.g., tables of sedative and narcotic equivalent doses). Long-term treatment of addictions is not discussed in this manual.

The information for this section was largely taken from Treatment of Drug Abuse Reactions. Med Lett Drug Ther 29:83–86, 1987. See also:

Millman RB (ed): Drug abuse and drug dependence. Psychiatr Update 5:120–227, 1986.

Lake CR (guest ed): Symposium on Clinical Pharmacology II. Psychiatr Clin North Am 7:657–756, 1984.

CANNABIS

Agents: marijuana and its derivatives; hashish, hash oil, THC (delta-9-tetrahydrocannabinol)

Specific agent, *street names*: marijuana, *pot, grass, weed, Mary Jane, THC, Acapulco gold, dope, sens similla*; marijuana cigarettes, *joint, reefer, roach, hit*; hashish, *hash, ganja, rope*

Intoxication Syndrome:
    Vital Signs—heart rate increased, blood pressure may show orthostatic drop
    Mental Status—anorexia, then increased appetite; euphoria, sensorium clear, dreamy or fantasy state, time-space distortion, rare hallucination; occasional panic or anxiety; with chronic use see amotivation, anergy
    Physical Examination—pupils normal size, slowed reaction to light, injected conjunctiva; in children see tachycardia, ataxia, pallor.

Management of Intoxication: No specific treatment is required. Anxiety symptoms may be treated with reassurance or benzodiazepines; psychotic symptoms may require haloperidol.

Withdrawal Syndrome: Nonspecific symptoms include anorexia, nausea, insomnia, restlessness, irritability, anxiety, and depression.

Management of Withdrawal: No specific intervention is required; long half-life of drug in body tissues leads to gradual withdrawal despite abrupt cessation of intake.

Medical Complications of Chronic Use: Impotence; may see respiratory problems with chronic smoking; susceptible persons may experience anxiety disorders or psychosis; amotivation syndrome.

CENTRAL NERVOUS SYSTEM DEPRESSANTS

Agents: alcohol, barbiturates, benzodiazepines, glutethimide, meprobamate, methaqualone, ethchlorvynol, ethinamate, chloral hydrate, methyprylon, paraldehyde

Specific agent, *street names:* barbiturates, *downers*; amobarbital, *blues;* chlordiazepoxide, *green and whites, roaches*; ethchlorvynol, *dyls*; methaqualone, *ludes, vit q, love drug*; secobarbital, *reds, pink ladies*; pentobarbital, *yellows*; seco- and amobarbital, *christmas trees*

Intoxication Syndrome:

   Vital Signs—respiration depressed, blood pressure decreased, shock in overdose

   Mental Status—drowsiness, confusion, coma, delirium

   Physical Examination—pupils dilated with glutethimide or in overdose, nystagmus, slowed reaction to light, tendon reflexes depressed, ataxia, slurred speech; convulsions or irritability with methaqualone, signs of anticholinergic toxicity with glutethimide, cardiac arrhythmias with chloral hydrate; overdosage results in hypoventilation, apnea, and death.

Management of Intoxication: For mild intoxication, observation will suffice, with treatment for withdrawal syndrome if it occurs. In overdose, maintain airway and treat with fluids if shock is present. Intubation followed by gastric lavage and instillation of activated charcoal may remove some of the drug.

Withdrawal Syndrome: Tremulousness, insomnia, sweating, fever, clonic blink reflex, anxiety, cardiovascular collapse, agitation, delirium, hallucinations, disorientation, seizure, and shock.

Management of Withdrawal Syndrome: Abrupt withdrawal of sedative agents can lead to life-threatening seizure or delirium. The dose should be tapered, or phenobarbital or chlordiazepoxide substituted in an appropriate dose to prevent withdrawal symptoms and then tapered (see the following table for substitute doses). Prolonged withdrawal reactions may occur with glutethimide or phenobarbital.

   Benzodiazepine withdrawal is particularly complicated because the withdrawal syndrome often imitates the anxiety syndromes for which these agents are prescribed. Gradual tapering of the dose over 10 days to several weeks is advised, particularly with long-acting benzodiazepines such as diazepam. Severe reactions have occurred after withdrawal of alprazolam, and gradual tapering of the dose is recommended.

Withdrawal from ethyl alcohol is similar to withdrawal from other sedative agents except that hepatic damage and malnutrition may exacerbate or cause delirium tremens, Wernicke's encephalopathy (characterized by delirium, ophthalmoplegia, and ataxia), or Korsakoff's psychosis. These serious complications can often be prevented by prompt intervention and management of the withdrawal syndrome, as described in the next section.

PROTOCOL FOR MANAGEMENT OF ETHYL ALCOHOL WITHDRAWAL

Severe Withdrawal Present or Predicted—Heavy daily drinking of some weeks' duration, history of severe withdrawal symptoms, hallucinations, seizures, or delirium tremens (DTs)

Chlordiazepoxide (Librium), 25–100 mg, orally; may be repeated every 1–2 hours as needed until symptoms are controlled, followed by

Chlordiazepoxide, 25–100 mg, every 2–4 hours for 24 hours as needed to keep symptoms controlled and patient mildly sedated,

Reduce and gradually withdraw chlordiazepoxide by approximately 20% per day; adjust schedule according to clinical situation; some patients can be withdrawn more quickly; lorazepam (Ativan) may be used in place of chlordiazepoxide if cirrhosis is present.

Moderate Withdrawal Predicted—Periodic heavy drinking or heavy daily drinking less than 1 week; no history of severe withdrawal

Chlordiazepoxide, 25–50 mg, every 2–4 hours as needed to control symptoms,

Then chlordiazepoxide, 25–50 mg, every 4 hours as needed

It is seldom necessary to use chlordiazepoxide for more than 3–5 days.

Mild Withdrawal Predicted—Minimal recent drinking; observe for withdrawal only

Be aware of possible other drug dependence and delayed withdrawal.

Do not administer chlordiazepoxide intravenously unless the patient is vomiting repeatedly. Intramuscular use is not recommended because absorption is unpredictable.

If the patient has a history of convulsions during withdrawal, take extra care in gradual withdrawal.

If adverse reaction to benzodiazepines, use phenobarbital and monitor closely.

Give multivitamin containing thiamine daily. If subclinical thiamine deficiency is suspected, give one 100-mg im injection of thiamine followed by 50 mg thiamine orally. Continue thiamine, 50 mg orally, for 10 days. With frank disorientation, ataxia, nystagmus, or ophthalmoplegia, give thiamine, 50 mg im **and** 50 mg iv; continue thiamine 50 or 100 mg, orally, for 10 days. Consider adding supplemental folate or magnesium. Intravenous thiamine must be given with dextrose solution.

PROTOCOL FOR MANAGEMENT OF WITHDRAWAL FROM SEDATIVE AGENTS OTHER THAN ALCOHOL

A pentobarbital tolerance test may be helpful in establishing approximate baseline dose requirements if the history is unclear or unreliable, or if the patient has consumed multiple agents with different potencies and half-lives. A protocol for the test follows this section.

Barbiturates—Use phenobarbital for withdrawal. Taper at approximately one sedative dose (30 mg) or 10% of first day's requirement each day after establishing the baseline dose that meets tolerance requirements.

Benzodiazepines—Use chlordiazepoxide or phenobarbital for withdrawal. Calculate equipotent dose; give in three or four divided doses per day; taper by 2.5%–10% per day based on patient's history of drug use and past withdrawal history (long-term use and history of complicated withdrawal suggest need for more gradual taper). Alprazolam may not be entirely cross-tolerant with other benzodiazepines; some authorities recommend taper of alprazolam itself. The use of clonazepam and carbamazepine has also been suggested.

Meprobamate—Consider taper of meprobamate itself because neither barbiturate nor benzodiazepine may fully substitute for its effects.

Others—Generally, phenobarbital can be substituted by equivalent sedative doses (see following table). This applies to chloral hydrate, ethchlorvynol, and methaqualone.

Medical Complications of Chronic Use: Risks of nonsterile injections and infectious complications may occur with intravenous use. Episodes of drug-induced sleep or coma may result in respiratory problems, nerve compression injuries, and accidents. Multiple medical problems may develop in chronic alcoholics, including nutritional deficiencies, megaloblastic anemia, psoriasis, gastritis, peptic ulcer, cirrhosis, pancreatitis, peripheral neuropathy, endocrinopathy, elevated triglycerides, and infectious diseases.

PENTOBARBITAL CHALLENGE TEST

Procedure should be performed only on inpatients with respiratory support staff and equipment available. Give 200 mg of pentobarbital orally to a fasting patient in resting state. The patient should be showing slight signs of withdrawal; do not give pentobarbital if the patient may have recently taken sedative agents.

Patient's condition 1 hour after test dose	Degree of tolerance	Estimated 24-hour pentobarbital requirement (mg)
Asleep, but arousable	Little or no tolerance	None
Drowsy, slurred speech, coarse nystagmus, Rombergism	Definite tolerance Marked intoxication	500–600
Comfortable, fine lateral nystagmus only drug effect	Marked tolerance Mild intoxication	800
No signs of drug effects, perhaps signs of abstinence persisting	Extreme tolerance No intoxication	1,000–1,200 or more

From Jackson AH, Shader RI: Guidelines for the withdrawal of narcotic and general depressant drugs. Dis Nerv Syst 34:162–166, 1973. By permission of Physicians Postgraduate Press.

WITHDRAWAL CONVERSIONS FOR SEDATIVE DRUGS

Generic name	Trade name	Dose (mg)	Withdrawal conversions
Benzodiazepines			
Alprazolam*	Xanax	0.25–0.5	
Chlordiaze-poxide	Librium	25	
Clonazepam	Klonopin	0.25	
Chlorazepate	Tranxene	15	
Diazepam	Valium	10	
Flurazepam	Dalmane	15	Chlordiazepoxide 25 mg
Halazepam	Paxipam	40	
Lorazepam	Ativan	1	
Oxazepam	Serax	30	
Prazepam	Centrax	10	
Temazepam	Restoril	15	
Triazolam	Halcion	0.25	
Barbiturates			
Amobarbital	Amytal	100	
Butabarbital	Many combinations	100	
Butalbital	Many combinations	100	Phenobarbital 30 mg
Pentobarbital	Nembutal	100	
Secobarbital	Seconal	100	
Others			
Chloral hydrate	Noctec	250	
Ethchlorvynol	Placidyl	200	Chlordiazepoxide 25 mg
Glutethimide	Doriden	250	or
Meprobamate†	Miltown, Equanil	400	Phenobarbital 30 mg
Methaqualone	Quaalude, Sopor	300	

*Withdrawal using alprazolam itself may be preferred to substitution of other drugs.
†Withdrawal using meprobamate itself may be preferred to substitution of other drugs.
Note: Care should be taken in the substitution of a long-acting drug for short- to medium-acting compounds to avoid excessive cumulative levels and toxicity. Daily "equivalent" doses should be divided and adjusted according to clinical response. Remember that patients' estimations of their own drug use may be quite inaccurate. The pentobarbital tolerance test may be useful.
Modified from Smith DE, Wesson DR: Benzodiazepine dependency syndromes. J Psychoactive Drugs 15:85–95, 1983.

CENTRAL NERVOUS SYSTEM STIMULANTS

Agents: cocaine, amphetamines, methylphenidate, phendimetrazine, phenylpropanolamine, diethylpropion, STP (2,5-dimethoxy-4-methylamphetamine), MDMA (3,4-methylenedioxymethamphetamine), bromo-DMA (4-bromo-2,5-dimethoxyamphetamine), amphetamine-like anti-obesity drugs

Specific agent, *street names*: cocaine, *coke, snow, blow, flake, crack, rock, crystal*; amphetamines, *speed, uppers, crank, whites, bennies, dexies, black beauties, white cross, meth, pep pills*; MDMA, *ecstasy*

Intoxication Syndrome, Overdose:
   Vital Signs—temperature elevation, increased heart rate, respiration shallow, blood pressure elevated.
   Mental Status—euphoria, disinhibition, grandiosity, sensorium hyperacute, paranoid ideation, mania, panic, hallucinations, delirium, impulsivity, irritability, hyperactivity, stereotypic movements
   Physical Examination—pupils dilated and sluggishly reactive, tendon reflexes hyperactive, cardiac arrhythmias, dry mouth, sweating; in overdose see tremors, convulsions, coma, stroke; with chronic use, erosion of nasal septum from "sniffing" cocaine, weight loss, evidence of malnutrition.

Management of Intoxication: Paranoia may be treated with haloperidol and seizures controlled with diazepam for cocaine and the amphetamines. Nitroprusside, phentolamine, or labetalol may be used to decrease blood pressure; cooling should be used to treat hyperthermia. Obtain electrocardiogram; cardiac dysrhythmias are common in acute intoxication.

Withdrawal Syndrome: Muscular aches, abdominal pain, chills, tremors, voracious hunger, anxiety, insomnia and periods of prolonged sleep, low energy, exhaustion, profound depression, and sometimes suicidal.

Management of Withdrawal: Generally no withdrawal medications are necessary. Cocaine, amphetamines, and amphetamine congeners may be stopped abruptly. Occasionally patients with chronic use of high-dose caffeine may experience discomfort (headache, dysphoria) that can be ameliorated by gradual withdrawal. Amantadine, carbamazepine, antidepressants, and bromocriptine have been suggested for relief of craving and dysphoria in cocaine addicts; tricyclic antidepressants are effective in relieving depression induced by withdrawal.

Medical Complications of Chronic Use: Weight loss, malnutrition; bronchiolitis obliterans organizing pneumonia from smoking "crack"; arrhythmias, myocardial infarction, and myocarditis; iv use carries hazards of nonsterile injections; sniffing cocaine results in necrosis of nasal septum.

HALLUCINOGENS

Agents: LSD (D-lysergic acid diethylamide), psilocybin, mescaline, PCP (phencyclidine)

Specific agent, *street names*: LSD, *acid, dot, microdot*; mescaline, *mushroom, shrooms, peyote, button*; phencyclidine, *angel dust, hog, crystal*

Intoxication Syndrome:
  Vital Signs—temperature elevated, heart rate increased, blood pressure elevated.
  Mental Status—euphoria, anxiety or panic, paranoia, sensorium may be clear, affect inappropriate, illusions, time and visual distortions, visual hallucinations, depersonalization; with PCP may see hypertensive encephalopathy.
  Physical Examination—pupils dilated (normal or small with PCP), tendon reflexes hyperactive; with PCP—nystagmus (vertical, horizontal, or circular), catatonia or extreme hyperactivity, drooling, blank stare, mutism, amnesia, analgesia, muscle rigidity, gait ataxia, impulsive or violent behavior, pressured speech.

Management of Intoxication: Most acute intoxications can be managed with calm reassurance in a quiet setting. PCP users may be particularly excitable and should be observed in a quiet area without interruption. Agitation may be treated with benzodiazepines; hyperthermia may occur and should be treated with rapid cooling. Haloperidol is preferred for treatment of persistent psychotic symptoms.

Withdrawal Syndrome: None.

Management of Withdrawal: None required after detoxification.

Medical Complications of Chronic Use: "Flashbacks," psychosis or anxiety syndromes may occur; use may induce lasting psychopathology in susceptible persons.

OPIATES

Agents: heroin, morphine, codeine, meperidine, methadone, hydromorphone, opium, pentazocine, propoxyphene, fentanyl, sufentanil

Specific agent, *street names*: heroin, *horse, h, junk, brown, smack, hard stuff, poppy, white stuff*; pentazocine, *Ts*

Intoxication Syndrome:
   Vital Signs—temperature decreased, respiration depressed, blood pressure decreased, sometimes shock.
   Mental Status—euphoria, stupor, coma.
   Physical Examination—pupils constricted (may be dilated with meperidine or in extreme hypoxia), nonreactive to light, reflexes diminished to absent, pulmonary edema, constipation, convulsions with propoxyphene or meperidine, cardiac arrhythmias with propoxyphene, coma, hypoventilation, apnea, death; depressant effects on respiration are additive with those of other central nervous system depressants.

Management of Intoxication: Naloxone will reverse apnea and coma caused by acute intoxication with heroin, morphine, codeine, and the synthetic narcotic analgesics (pentazocine may be an exception). Naloxone will not reverse pulmonary edema. An initial intravenous or intramuscular dose of 0.4–2 mg of naloxone can be repeated at 2- to 3-minute intervals until clinical response is adequate, followed by an intravenous infusion of two-thirds of the total dose each hour. The patient should be closely monitored as naloxone has a much shorter half-life than most opioids; overdosage of methadone, which has a 24-hour half-life, may require carefully titrated doses of naloxone over 72 hours. Excessive doses of naloxone can precipitate abrupt withdrawal in opiate-dependent patients and should be avoided.

Withdrawal Syndrome: Pupils dilated, pulse rapid, gooseflesh, lacrimation, rhinorrhea, abdominal cramps, diarrhea, muscle jerks, flu-like syndrome, vomiting, tremulousness, yawning, anxiety, and insomnia; sleep and mood disturbance after acute detoxification may be present for several weeks. A table of withdrawal stages is included with this section.

Management of Withdrawal: Withdrawal, although extremely uncomfortable, is generally life threatening only for newborns. Pregnant women should be maintained on methadone or withdrawn slowly. Most opiate-dependent patients can be managed with oral methadone; establish baseline requirements by history and objective evidence of recent use, then adjust the dose empirically by objective signs of withdrawal or intoxication. A table of methadone equivalents is included with this section. If baseline dose is unknown, 15–20 mg of methadone may be given and the patient's condition observed; 40 mg in 24 hours will prevent withdrawal in most patients. Taper the baseline dose at 10%–20% per day depending on past history of drug use and withdrawal complications. Clonidine has been used as an alternative to methadone, in a dosage of 2 mg per day in divided doses (or 5 µg/kg per dose).

Special Considerations in Opiate Withdrawal: The use of methadone management for withdrawal from some of the potent, short-acting opiates may not be necessary (e.g., fentanyl and butorphanol); time of last use, route of entry, pharmacokinetics of the compound, dose, and duration of use should be considered. Withdrawal from pentazocine, propoxyphene, and butorphanol if required, is best handled by taper of the drug itself. Propoxyphene napsylate may be used to withdraw from itself or from propoxyphene hydrochloride (100 mg propoxyphene napsylate = 65 mg propoxyphene hydrochloride).

Medical Complications of Chronic Use: Illegal opioids may be adulterated with quinine, lactose, mannitol, or other drugs and may be contaminated with bacteria, fungi, viruses, or particulate matter. Pulmonary emboli, myocarditis, endocarditis, and sepsis may result from intravenous use. Sharing intravenous equipment exposes users to blood-borne infections such as hepatitis and AIDS. Use of MPTP (1-methyl-4-phenyl-1,2,3,6-tetrahydropyridine), a contaminant found in illicit preparations of meperidine, has resulted in permanent parkinsonism and death.

NARCOTIC WITHDRAWAL STAGES

Abstinence signs* in sequential appearance after last dose of narcotic in patients with well-established habits of parenteral use

Grades of abstinence	Signs (observed in cool room, patient uncovered or under only a sheet)	Hours after last dose						
		Morphine	Heroin	Meperidine	Dihydromorphinone	Codeine	Methadone
Grade 0	Craving for drug Anxiety	6	4	2–3	2–3	8	12
Grade 1	Yawning Perspiration Lacrimation Rhinorrhea	14	8	4–6	4–5	24	34–48
Grade 2	Increase in above signs plus: Mydriasis Gooseflesh (piloerection) Tremors (muscle twitches) Hot and cold flashes Aching bones and muscles Anorexia	16	12	8–12	7	48	48–72

Grade 3	Increased intensity of above plus: Insomnia Increased blood pressure Increased temperature Increased respiratory rate and depth Increased pulse rate Restlessness Nausea	24–36	18–24	16	12	… …
Grade 4	Increased intensity of above plus: Febrile facies Position—curled up on hard surface Vomiting Weight loss (5 lb daily) Spontaneous ejaculation or orgasm Hemoconcentration— leukocytosis, eosinopenia, increased blood sugar	36–48	24–36	…	16	… …

Note: Racemorphan (Dromoran) and levorphanol (Levo-Dromoran), although 3 times and 6 times, respectively, as strong as morphine sulfate, show same time curve as morphine sulfate, as do paregoric, laudanum, and hydrochlorides of opium alkaloids (Pantopon), depending on their relative content of morphine.

*Not all signs are necessary to diagnose any particular grade.

From Blachly PH: Management of the opiate abstinence syndrome. Am J Psychiatry 122:742–744, 1966. By permission of the American Psychiatric Association.

METHADONE WITHDRAWAL EQUIVALENTS

1 mg methadone is equivalent to:

   3 mg morphine sulfate
   1–2 mg heroin
   20 mg meperidine (Demerol)
   0.5 mg dihydromorphinone (Dilaudid)
   3–5 mg oxycodone (Percodan)
   4 mg hydrochlorides of opium alkaloids (Pantopon)
   0.5 mg levorphanol (Levo-Dromoran)
   7–8 ml paregoric (contains 0.4 morphine per ml, but less than
      half absorbed)
   0.3 ml laudanum (1% tincture of morphine)

Modified from Blachly PH: Management of the opiate abstinence syndrome. Am J Psychiatry 122:742–744, 1966.

VOLATILE INHALANTS

Agents: nitrous oxide; amyl-, butyl-, isobutyl nitrites; toluene; 1,2-dichloropropane (spot-remover compounds); acetone; bromo-chlorodifluoromethane (BCF); gasoline; 1,1,1-trichlorethane, perchloroethylene, trichloroethylene (used in typewriter correction fluids, glue, and fabric stain protectors); methylene chloride

Street names: rush, poppers, locker room

Intoxication Syndrome: varies with agent used
   Vital Signs—heart rate increased, respiration may be increased and shallow, blood pressure decreased.
   Mental Status—transient euphoria, dizziness, confusion, delirium, hallucinations, somnolence, encephalopathy.
   Physical Examination—pupil normal or dilated; other physical findings reflect major organ toxicities; in severe intoxications see renal or hepatic damage with resulting electrolyte disturbances, renal tubular acidosis, renal failure, disseminated intravascular coagulation; neurologic complications include peripheral neuropathies, encephalopathy, ataxia, cerebellar dysfunction, headache, seizures; some agents cause myocardiopathy, arrhythymias, sudden death.

Management of Intoxication: Support major organ systems as necessary and monitor for changes in vital signs or mental status that may reflect complications.

Withdrawal: Withdrawal syndromes appear to be rare.

Management of Withdrawal: None required after acute detoxification.

Medical Complications of Chronic Use: Inhalation of amyl-, butyl-, or isobutyl nitrite causes methemoglobinemia; inhalation of methylene chloride may cause carbon monoxide poisoning; inhalation of leaded gasoline causes lead toxicity; toxic effects on major organs may be permanent.

ANTICHOLINERGICS

Agents: atropine, belladonna, henbane, scopolamine, trihexyphenidyl, benztropine mesylate, procyclidine, propantheline bromide, jimson weed seed

Specific agents, *street names*: belladonna, *donna*

Intoxication Syndrome:
   Vital Signs—temperature elevated, heart rate increased, blood pressure may be decreased.
   Mental Status—drowsiness or coma, sensorium clouded, amnesia, disorientation, visual hallucinations, body image alterations, confusion, sometimes restlessness, paranoia, excitement.
   Physical Examination—pupils dilated and nonreactive; decreased bowel sounds; flushed, dry skin and mucous membranes; violent behavior; seizures. With propantheline, may see circulatory failure, respiratory failure, paralysis, coma.

Management of Intoxication: Careful monitoring and symptomatic support will usually suffice; physostigmine should be reserved for signs of life-threatening anticholinergic toxicity (uncontrolled seizures, respiratory depression, or severe hypertension).

Withdrawal Syndrome: Gastrointestinal discomfort and dysmotility and musculoskeletal symptoms occur.

Management of Withdrawal Syndrome: No specific management required after acute detoxification.

Medical Complications of Chronic Use: May see increased risk of glaucoma, gastrointestinal dysmotility, or complications of urinary retention.

ELECTROCONVULSIVE THERAPY (ECT)

GENERAL CONSIDERATIONS

1. The National Institute of Mental Health Consensus Development Conference on ECT found that ECT is useful for depression, acute mania, and some schizophrenic syndromes.

2. Unilateral stimulus to the nondominant hemisphere is preferred in order to minimize post-ECT confusion and memory loss, but some patients respond better to a bilateral stimulus.

3. Increased seizure threshold may occur with advancing age, prior ECT, and anticonvulsant therapy. Unilateral lead placement is associated with a lower seizure threshold, but a higher-energy stimulus may be required for therapeutic efficacy.

4. In general, use of psychotropic medications, especially lithium, should be minimized or avoided during ECT.

5. Conditions requiring special consideration prior to the use of ECT. (With adequate precautions there are no absolute contraindications to the use of ECT.)

   ECT generally contraindicated:

   Increased intracranial pressure

   Space-occupying intracranial lesion

   Recent head injury

   Extra precautions required:

   Hypo- or hyperkalemia

   Porphyria

   Glaucoma

   Recent myocardial infarction

   Recent cerebrovascular accident

   Cardiac arrhythmia

   Coronary artery disease

   Uncontrolled hypertension

   Untreated venous thrombosis

   Other medications or conditions that might prolong seizure or complicate anesthesia and muscle relaxation

6. Post-ECT agitation may respond to a short-acting benzodiazepine. This may be administered intravenously after treatment. For headaches, prescribe mild analgesic; for nausea, prescribe

dimenhydrinate or other antiemetic; for prolonged seizure, administer diazepam 5 mg iv by slow infusion.
7. Legislative regulation of ECT varies from state to state; physicians should familiarize themselves with local laws regarding informed consent and administration of ECT to voluntary, involuntary, incompetent, and juvenile patients.

See also:
Abrams R: Electroconvulsive Therapy. New York, Oxford University Press, 1988.
Rose RM, Pincus HA (section eds): Electroconvulsive therapy. Rev Psychiatry 7:431–528, 1988.

ELECTROCONVULSIVE THERAPY (ECT) PROCEDURE GUIDELINES

ECT should be administered by trained personnel with necessary equipment and personnel on site for cardiopulmonary resuscitation or treatment of complications that may arise.

Prior to Treatment:
1. Patient should undergo medical and psychiatric evaluations, including history, general physical and neurologic examinations, electrocardiogram, and other laboratory tests as indicated. Consider obtaining a pretreatment electroencephalogram and brain imaging study (CT or MRI).
2. Explain ECT to patient and family; obtain informed consent from patient, family, and/or guardian.
3. Discontinue medications if possible. In general, monoamine oxidase inhibitors should be stopped 2 weeks prior to treatment; lithium should be stopped with time for a washout period; severe hypertension should be controlled. Benzodiazepines will decrease the seizure duration and increase the seizure threshold. If benzodiazepines are required between treatments, those with short half-lives and no active metabolites should be used.
4. Patient should have no oral intake for 8–12 hours prior to the procedure.
5. Anticholinergic drug (e.g., glycopyrrolate or atropine) is administered to decrease secretions.
6. Patient should empty bladder and remove dentures.

During Treatment:

7. A peripheral intravenous line is placed; sedative anesthetic (e.g., methohexital or pentothal) is administered followed by muscle relaxant (e.g., succinylcholine).

8. Electrocardiogram, blood pressure, and pulse are monitored throughout; 100% oxygen is administered with positive pressure bag. Transdermal oxygen monitoring may be performed.

9. Electrodes are placed bifrontotemporally for bilateral stimulus, or frontotemporally on the nondominant hemisphere for unilateral stimulus. Unilateral placement is generally preferred to minimize confusion but bilateral is more effective in some conditions.

10. Enough electrical stimulus is applied to induce a generalized seizure. A brief pulsed stimulus is associated with fewer cognitive deficits than the traditional sine-wave stimulus.

11. The seizure is monitored and duration is recorded. Seizure monitoring may be via electroencephalogram or by inflating a blood pressure cuff above systolic pressure on a distal extremity site prior to administration of the muscle relaxant (succinylcholine). In unilateral ECT, place cuff on the same side as the lateral electrode to demonstrate generalized spread of the seizure to both cerebral hemispheres.

12. Six treatments are usually the minimum required for affective disorders or psychosis. Treatments are usually given every other day or thrice weekly.

After Treatment:

13. In the patient's chart, record the seizure duration, electrical stimulus applied, type and dose of drugs administered, and patient's condition.

14. The patient is monitored closely after the treatment until breathing is adequate without support.

Modified from Electroconvulsive therapy. JAMA 254:2103–2108, 1985.
See also: Frankel FH (chairperson): Electroconvulsive Therapy: Report of the Task Force on Electroconvulsive Therapy (Task Force Report 14). Washington, DC, American Psychiatric Association, 1978.

SAMPLE ELECTROCONVULSIVE THERAPY (ECT) CONSENT FORM

This sample consent form for ECT is included as a guide to facilitate discussion with patients.

I, _____,
(Physician)

recommend electroconvulsive therapy for treatment of your current psychiatric problem.

Electroconvulsive therapy, or ECT, has been used since 1938 to treat certain psychiatric disorders such as major depression with melancholia with or without psychotic features and with or without suicidal intent, mania, and schizophrenia—especially catatonic schizophrenia. Occasionally, patients with other psychiatric disorders unresponsive to medication, such as PCP-induced psychosis, and patients with psychiatric disorders who are too medically ill to tolerate medication side effects benefit from ECT.

The treatments occur three times a week on Monday, Wednesday, and Friday (unless the severity of symptoms necessitates an increase in the frequency of treatments to every day), and they last for 2–6 weeks, depending on the nature of the patient's illness. The treatments occur in the morning and last only a few minutes. Once the treatment is complete, patients are observed in a post-ECT monitoring room until they are fully alert and ready to return to their room, eat breakfast, and resume normal activities.

When one enters the treatment suite for treatment, there will be an anesthetist, a psychiatric nurse, and a psychiatric physician to provide the treatment. A needle will be placed in the vein to inject anesthetic agents for the treatment. These agents include a preanesthetic drug, a barbiturate for inducing sleep, and succinylcholine for relaxing muscles. Oxygen is administered prior to the treatment.

During the anesthetic preparation, the psychiatric nurse and psychiatric physician will prepare the patient for the actual treatment. This includes placement of electrodes on the patient's head to deliver the treatment and a testing of the machine to ensure proper functioning prior to the actual administration of treatment. Once the patient is asleep from the anesthetics, the treatment is given.

Common risks include drowsiness and confusion following the procedure, memory loss for the event, and transient headache or muscle aches. Uncommon but potentially serious risks include complications of anesthesia, prolonged memory loss, bone fractures, and death in 1 of every 10,000–40,000 patients treated with this procedure.

Finally, you have the right to withdraw from treatment with ECT at any time. However, early discontinuation of treatment may precipitate a relapse of the psychiatric problem(s) for which ECT was recommended.

I, _____,
(Patient or Guardian)

on _____ , have read this
(Date)

description of ECT and/or have had these descriptions explained to

me by _____,
(Physician)

and I agree to proceed with this form of therapy.

In addition to the above, the reasons for ECT treatment and potential benefits as well as alternate forms of treatment—with their risks and benefits—must be discussed with the patient and guardians. The risks of not treating the condition must also be explained. These items are not covered in the consent form because they must be individualized according to the patient's psychiatric and medical condition.

FORMAT FOR HOSPITAL DISMISSAL SUMMARY

A concise final "progress" note summarizes the patient's hospitalization. This note frequently serves as a summary for follow-up treatment and for hospital utilization and third-party payer review. Confidential disclosures should be avoided in this setting. The following format is useful.

Name; Patient Identification Number; Source of Referral
Admission Date; Dismissal Date; Physician's Name
Chief Complaint: As per patient; reason for referral
Present Psychiatric Illness
Pertinent Medical History
Initial Mental Status Examination
Physical Examination: Positive findings
Laboratory and Imaging Data; Psychologic Testing
Consultations: Include date, physician, service, findings, and
    recommendations
Treatment and Course: Psychotherapy, pharmacotherapy, electro-
    convulsive therapy, other
Condition and Disposition at Dismissal: Include disability status or
    return-to-work recommendations, plan for follow-up, means to
    contact patient. Note specifically which conditions resolved dur-
    ing the hospital stay and which persisted at dismissal. Prognosis
    may be included here
Dismissal Diagnoses: DSM-III-R preferred, include organic diag-
    noses on Axis III
Dismissal Medications: Including amounts prescribed
Letters: Full names, complete addresses, and notation as to relation-
    ship to patient (i.e., referring family physician; new psychiatrist
    who will see patient in follow-up; letter to patient)

TELEPHONE NUMBERS

One of the most useful sections of our original handbook was the compilation of telephone numbers of the local mental health network. We offer some suggestions below.

Hospital Based	Name	Number
Attending M.D.		
Pager	_____	_____
Home	_____	_____
Office	_____	_____
On-call pager	_____	_____
Closed Psychiatry Unit	_____	_____
Open Psychiatry Unit	_____	_____
Adolescent Unit	_____	_____
Hospital Operator	_____	_____
Emergency Room	_____	_____
Pharmacy	_____	_____
Legal Advisor	_____	_____
Preadmission Certification	_____	_____

Clinic Based		
Clinic Operator	_____	_____
Appointment Secretary	_____	_____
Attending Physician's Secretary	_____	_____
Clinical Psychologist	_____	_____
Office of	Dr. _____	_____
Office of	Dr. _____	_____

Local Mental Health		
County Mental Health Center	_____	_____
State Mental Hospital	_____	_____
Veterans Administration Hospital	_____	_____
County Social Services	_____	_____
County Social Worker	_____	_____

	Name	Number
County Courthouse		
Law Enforcement		
Public School Counselor		
Half-Way House		
Medical Examiner		
Detoxification Center		
Crisis Center		
Alcoholics Anonymous Information		
Women's Shelter		
Sheltered Workshop		

Reimbursement

Insurance Information		
Health Maintenance Organization		
Medical Assistance		
County		
State		

Professional Organizations

American Academy of Child and Adolescent Psychiatry		
American Psychiatric Association		

Other Professional Organizations

State Psychiatric Association		
Local Psychiatric Association		

Other

INDEX